Implantology in General Dental Practice

Quintessentials of Dental Practice – 4

Implantology in General Dental Practice

By
Lloyd Searson
Martin Gough
Ken Hemmings

Editor-in-Chief: Nairn H F Wilson

Quintessence Publishing Co. Ltd.
London, Berlin, Chicago, Paris, Milan, Barcelona, Istanbul,
São Paulo, Tokyo, New Delhi, Moscow, Prague, Warsaw

SEP 2 1 2005

British Library Cataloguing-in Publication Data

Searson, Lloyd J. J.
Implantology in general dental practice. – (Quintessentials of dental practice ; 4)
1. Dental implants
I. Title II. Gough, Martin III. Hemmings, Kenneth W.
617.6´9

ISBN 1850970548

ISBN 1-85097-054-8

Foreword

Implantology is one of the most exciting and dynamic aspects of modern dentistry. Developments in implant systems and techniques have transformed prosthodontics at all levels. Practitioners not yet into implants, and those whose knowledge and understanding in this field are limited, will find this addition to the *Quintessentials of Dental Practice* series to be an excellent acquisition. Apart from dispelling much of the mystique that has built up around implants and their use, this book provides an abundance of practical guidance of immediate relevance to everyday clinical practice. As with all the volumes in the *Quintessential* series, this book is not intended to be a comprehensive tome on the subject; it is a succinct, easy-to-read, well illustrated overview of key points and essential guidance.

Whether this book is your starting point, springboard to more comprehensive texts or aid to reinforce existing knowledge and understanding of implantology, it should not disappoint. Indeed, I would be dismayed if it did not stimulate its readers to offer at least some, or hopefully more, implant-based forms of treatment to their patients. Do you owe it to your patients, professional development and practice to purchase this volume and find the few hours needed to read it from cover to cover? If you do, it will be time and money well spent.

Nairn Wilson
Editor-in-Chief

Preface

Implants are now a recognised treatment for partially dentate and edentulous patients. This book is based on our joint experiences over 15 years working in the Restorative Department at the Eastman Dental Hospital and in private practice. Our aim is to provide general dental practitioners with a concise introduction to dental implantology and enable them to discuss implants as a treatment option with patients.

Lloyd Searson
Martin Gough
Ken Hemmings

Acknowledgements

We would like to thank the many people who have helped us put together all the information included. Particularly we would like to thank Dr David Gallacher, Radiology department, Guy's and St Thomas' Hospital, and Dr Anthony Reynolds, Image Diagnostic Technology Ltd, The London Imaging Centre. Our special thanks go to all the highly skilled technical teams at the Eastman Dental Hospital.

Contents

Chapter 1
History and Development of Dental Implants

Aim

The aim of this chapter is to familiarise the reader with the history and development of dental implants and with relevant terminology and implant characteristics.

Outcome

After reading this chapter the reader should have an understanding of dental implants, their design and characteristics and the various components that are used in implant dentistry.

Introduction

Tooth loss as a result of disease, trauma, failure to develop and the adverse consequence of partial dentures is common. It is not surprising, therefore, that the history of tooth replacement has been long and multifaceted. Depending on the degree of edentulism, several treatment options are available, including:

- no replacement
- removable partial dentures
- complete dentures
- conventional or adhesive bridgework
- implant-supported prostheses
- transplantation.

The management of edentulism poses a challenge to the practitioner. Evidence from ancient civilisations has shown throughout history that man has tried to replace missing and lost teeth with various materials, including carved ivory, wood and bone. At times, natural teeth were extracted from paupers and casualties of war to replace missing teeth in the wealthy.

It was not until the 19th century that experiments using different materials and designs of appliances to replace missing teeth were reported in the dental literature. Attempted replacements ranged from the use of root-form gold implants placed into sockets to iridium-platinum basket-type endosteal implants with screws.

Before the 1950s implant placement was more of an art form than a science. It was not until the late 1970s/early 1980s that the use of dental implants became more scientific and implantology was recognised by the academic community.

The two main research groups responsible for the underpinning science were Brånemark and co-workers in the late 1960s, and Schroeder and co-workers in the mid-1970s. Both research groups established that direct contact exists between bone and dental titanium implants and that this contact results in the clinical stability of an implant during loading. For this mode of anchorage, Brånemark and co-workers coined the term "osseointegration" in 1967. Osseointegration is the direct structural and functional connection between ordered living bone and the surface of a load-carrying implant.

Osseointegration heralded a fundamental scientific shift in thinking, previous implants having tended to develop a fibrous attachment that, it was hoped, could serve the same purpose as the periodontal ligament. The periodontal ligament is a specialised structure that serves as an effective attachment mechanism, a shock absorber and a sensory organ. Furthermore, the periodontal ligament is capable of mediating bone remodelling, allowing tooth movement. Previous non-integrating forms of implants may have been anchored to bone by means of a surrounding sheath of pseudo periodontal ligament, but this fibrous sheath was a poorly differentiated layer of scar tissue. In most cases, loading and gradual widening of this led to loosening of the implant and subsequent implant failure (Fig 1-1).

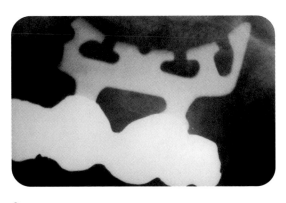

Fig 1-1 Radiograph of blade implant showing implant failure.

Implants

There are three types of implants available:
• subperiosteal
• transosseous
• endosseous.

Subperiosteal
This type of implant consists of a non-osteointegrated framework that rests on the surface bone of the mandible or maxilla. The framework is positioned beneath the mucosa with, typically, a number of posts penetrating the mucosa to support an overdenture.

Subperiosteal implants were originally introduced in the 1940s and served patients well for many years. Unfortunately, problems experienced included infection, exteriorisation by the downgrowth of epithelium and damage to the underlying bone. In some cases the subperiosteal implant would submerge into the bone, making it extremely difficult to remove (Fig 1-2).

Transosseous
The transmandibular staple is the most used form of transosseous implant, consisting of a gold plate fitted to the lower border of the mandible and posts placed directly through the mandible to provide support for some form of denture. This approach was suitable only for the mandible. Although some reports show good results over periods of up to 10 years, the use of transosseous implants has been largely discontinued (Fig 1-3 and Fig 1-4).

Endosseous
These implants can be placed in the maxilla or mandible through an intra-

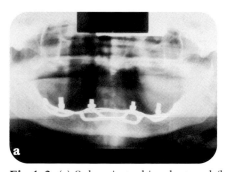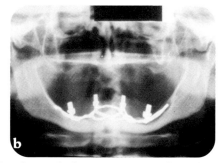

Fig 1-2 (a) Subperiosteal implant and (b) radiograph showing extensive bone loss around a subperiosteal implant.

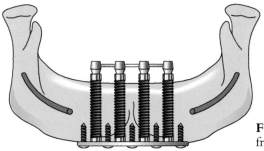

Fig 1-3 Transosseous implant frame.

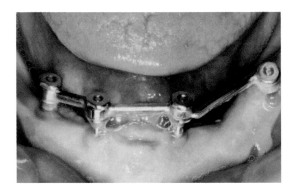

Fig 1-4 Intraoral view of transmandibular staple implant.

oral incision in the mucoperiosteum. The shapes and construction of endosseous implants have varied over the years, but the past two decades have seen the most dynamic developments. The clinician may be bewildered by the variety of implant shapes and designs available. However, various groups have developed certain criteria that aid the selection of implant systems. For example, Albrektsson and co-workers (1986) proposed the following criteria for a successful implant:

- The freestanding implant should be rigid clinically.
- Radiographic examination does not reveal any peri–implant radiolucency.
- In clinical service radiographic vertical bone loss is less than 0.2mm each year.
- Absence of signs or symptoms of failure, including pain, infection, neuropathies, paraesthesia or violation of anatomical structures.
- A success rate of 85% at the end of a five-year observation period and 80% at the end of a 10-year period.

Factors Influencing Implant Osseointegration

Osseointegration is a union between bone and the implant surface. It can be measured histologically as the proportion of the total implant surface that is in direct contact with bone. Different levels of bone contact may occur with implants of different materials. There are a number of factors that may influence the degree of osseointegration, relating to one of three parameters:

• implant design
• host site
• surgical technique.

Implant Design

Most contemporary dental implants are made of commercially pure titanium, which has been shown to have excellent biocompatibility. Titanium is a light metal. When exposed to air, a surface oxide is rapidly formed. This layer of oxide determines the biological response. Commercially pure titanium is also highly resistant to corrosion. Other metals have been used for osseointegration, including zirconium, gold and titanium-aluminium-vanadium alloys. These alloys may strengthen the implant but have been shown to have relatively poor bone-to-implant contact.

Implant design has a great influence on the stability and subsequent function of the implant in bone. The main parameters are implant shape, implant

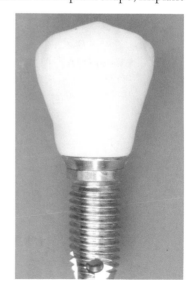

Fig 1-5 Screw-shaped implant with abutment and final prosthesis in position.

length, implant diameter and surface characteristics. Root-form implants, such as screws and cylinders, are the dominating implant designs today. Screw implants are considered to be superior to cylindrical ones in terms of initial stability and resistance to compression and tension stresses under loading (Fig 1-5).

Implant Length
Research findings have shown that shorter implants fail more often than longer implants. Implant length varies from 6-20mm. The most common lengths employed are between 8- 15mm. It is good practice to use the longest implant that can be safely placed, with, wherever possible bicortical stability. Clearly, certain anatomical limitations exist, for example, in the posterior mandible behind the mental foramen.

Implant Diameters
The diameter of most implants falls within the range of 3.3-6mm. Narrow diameter implants can be used in small spaces. Larger diameter implants may be used, in particular in posterior areas of the mouth and where there is poor quality bone.

Surface Characteristics
It has been suggested that the quality of osseointegration is related to the physical and chemical nature of the surface of the implant. Surface characteristics may be altered by several means including:
- Machining - the surface is produced by precision milling with no subsequent finishing.
- Plasma-spraying - spraying with molten titanium modifies and increases the effective surface area of the implant.
- Machine grit-blasting - the implant surface is roughened by grit-blasting with titanium oxide particles.
- Acid-etching - the implant surface is chemically etched to increase the thickness of the oxide layer.
- Sand-blasting and acid-etching – sand-blasting followed by acid-etching to substantially increase surface area.
- Anodisation - the implant surface is electrically treated to increase the thickness of the oxide layer.
- Coating - the implant surface is coated with calcium phosphate hydroxyapatite to produce a so-called bioactive surface to enhance bone-to-implant contact.
- Increasing surface roughness increases the bone-to-implant contact area and, in turn, osseointegration (Fig 1-6). The ideal surface morphology

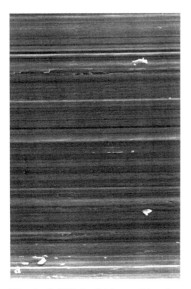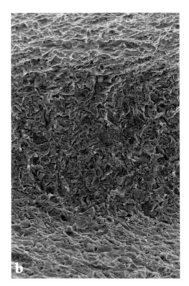

Fig 1-6 SEM of (a) machined surface implant and (b) ti-blasted surface (Courtesy of Prof. Neil Meredith).

is yet to be determined. Short-term studies support the use of rougher surfaces, but long-term results are required to confirm such findings. The current trend is towards increased surface roughness, either from blasting or etching.

The Host Site
Bone Factors
There are differences in the anatomy of the bone of the maxilla and the mandible. As a consequence, a higher ratio of compact to cancellous bone exists in the mandible. Bone density has been found to be an important factor in the initial stability and prevention of micromovement of the implant. Determination of bone quantity will be considered in subsequent chapters. Assessment of bone quality is more difficult. Sectional tomograms and computed tomography scans provide an indication of medullary bone density.

From a clinical point of view, the quality of bone can be assessed during surgery, based on subjective feel and by assessing cutting resistance during drilling, tapping and placement of the implant. The initial stability can be quantified using resonance frequency analysis (RFA), which is a non-invasive method to evaluate implants stability.

General Health
A review of the literature indicates that patients with a variety of systemic conditions may be successfully treated with dental implants. As with all patients undergoing a surgical procedure, advice may be required from the patient's physician.

Age
Implant placement is not recommended in young patients prior to completion of growth as the implants may end up in infraocclusion. It is widely recommended to wait until the patient is at least 17 to 18 years old. Completion of growth is usually earlier in females than males.

Although wound-healing in the elderly is slower than in young individuals, given reduced local vascularity and bone density, there is no upper age limit to implant placement, as long as the patient is fit and able to undergo the necessary surgery.

Smoking
Smoking is a well-established risk to general health and a factor in periodontitis. Other adverse effects of smoking include systemic vasoconstriction, reduced blood flow and increased platelet aggregation. These effects contribute to reasons why dental implants have approximately twice the failure rate in smokers compared to non-smokers. All implant patients should be encouraged to stop smoking or to at least stop smoking for several weeks before and after the surgical placement of implants.

Radiotherapy
Previous radiotherapy to the jaws for the treatment of malignant disease will result in endartertis with impaired bone-healing. Success rates of dental implants are lower in patients with a history of radiotherapy compared to non-irradiated patients. Patients with a history of radiotherapy should be referred to specialist centres, which may be able to provide, for example, hyperbaric oxygen therapy to improve the chance of success.

Surgical Technique
Surgical Experience
Clinical experience and surgical skill have been shown to have an impact on implant success rates. It is therefore imperative that those wishing to place implants receive sufficient training to become competent in all relevant procedures.

Operating Conditions
Implant surgery should be performed under highly controlled conditions. Contamination of the implant surface during surgical placement should be avoided. Possible sources of contamination from non-titanium surgical instruments and the patient's saliva will, in all probability, have a negative effect on osseointegration.

Incision Technique
A number of different incision types have been advocated, and these will be considered in the chapter on surgical technique.

Drilling Technique
Frictional heat during any phase of the drilling procedure will cause a rise in temperature. The critical time/temperature parameter for bone tissue necrosis is around 47°C for one minute. The generation of heat can be kept to a minimum by the use of sharp drills, slow drill speeds, graduated drill sizes and copious water-cooling.

Healing and Loading Times
The time from implant insertion to functional loading may be classified into the following categories:
• delayed loading – four to six months
• early loading – one to two months
• immediate loading.

Delayed loading - this tried and tested approach involves the implant not being loaded following placement until approximately six months in the maxilla and four months in the mandible. The difference in timing is primarily related to the difference in bone quality between the maxilla and mandible.

Early loading - a number of implant systems with roughened thread designs are considered to be appropriate for early loading within six weeks of implant placement. Such implants should only be placed in good quality bone and under favourable circumstances.

Immediate loading - in exceptional cases it has been suggested that it may be possible to consider the immediate loading of implants. Factors such as initial implant fit, quality and quantity of available bone, length and diameter of implant, occlusal factors and experience of the operator should be taken into consideration.

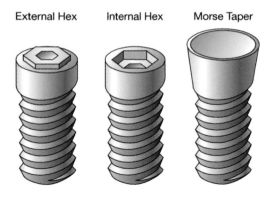

External Hex   **Internal Hex**   **Morse Taper**

Fig 1-7 External and internal hex and Morse taper connectors.

Implant Componentry

The clinician may be bewildered by the variety of implant systems available. In making a choice, various aspects of the implant design, implant to abutment connection, instrumentation and the final prosthesis should be considered.

Implant Design
The majority of dental implants are made from commercially pure titanium and are cylindrical in design. A thread increases surface area, enhances initial stability and redistributes functional forces. It is now accepted that a modified surface will increase surface area, improve sheer strength, enhance osseointegration and shorten treatment times.

Dental implants are available with both external and internal connections, which aid in the attachment of the abutment or final prosthesis. The external connection is most commonly a "hexagonal" feature. Internal connections are available in different designs, including an internal hex or Morse taper (Fig 1-7).

Implant to Abutment Connection and Implant to Final Prostheses Connection
A final prosthesis may be connected to the implant in several ways (Fig 1-8):
• screw retained direct to the implant
• screw retained to the abutment
• lateral/horizontal screw retained to abutment
• cement retained to abutment.

Screw-Retained Prostheses Connection
Advantages of this approach include:

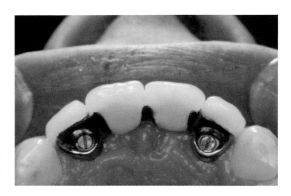

Fig 1-8 Palatal view of a screw-retained partial prosthesis.

- retrievability
- machined-component interface
- no cement breakdown or extrusion from joint at time of placement
- screw loosening may warn of mechanical overload.

Disadvantages include:
- compromised aesthetics with screw access to implant or abutment being visible on occlusal surfaces
- increased bulk of cingulum in anterior teeth
- achieving passive fit requires considerable technical skill (Fig 1-9).

Cement-Retained Prostheses Connection
Advantages of cement-retained prostheses include:
- improved aesthetics in the absence of occlusal access holes
- accuracy of fit not as critical as with screw retention
- clinical and laboratory techniques similar to conventional crown and bridgework.

Disadvantages include:
- retrievability may be difficult
- increased cost of production given the need for a secondary casting
- excess cement maybe extruded into soft tissues (Figs 1-10).

Abutment
A dental abutment is typically a machined or custom-made component that connects the final prosthesis to the implant. The abutment may be made from a variety of materials.

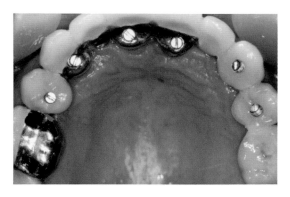

Fig 1-9 Customised abutments for a cement-retained partial prosthesis.

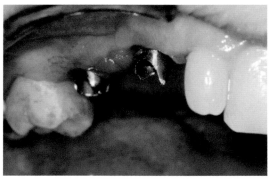

Fig 1-10 Extensive full arch screw-retained maxilla prosthesis – displaying the ease of retrievability.

A machined abutment is typically manufactured from titanium, gold or ceramic. The advantages of this type of abutment are that it is simple to use, requires minimal chairside and laboratory time and has a predictable precision fit and good retention.

A customised abutment may be prepable, custom-made in the laboratory or computer-aided design – computer-aided manufacture (CAD-CAM) designed. A prepable abutment is generally supplied by the manufacturer as a blank in titanium or ceramic to be modified by the clinician at the chairside or by the dental technician on the master model. Customisation in the laboratory typically involves waxing to the required design and casting. A CAD-CAM-designed abutment is produced with specialised computer software and a milling machine.

The selection and use of an abutment is determined by a number of factors, including implant angulation and orientation, depth of soft tissue from implant body to gingival cuff, aesthetic demands, interocclusal space and preference for a cement or screw- retained prosthesis.

Choice of Implants System

A survey of dental practitioners providing implants revealed the following features to be important in selecting implant systems:
• fulfilling national and international standards
• documented clinical success
• commercially pure titanium
• cylindrical, threaded implant design
• both submerged and non-submerged protocol
• a modified roughened surface
• a universal implant for all bone types
• a universal protocol for immediate and early loading
• various lengths and diameters
• a standardised abutment implant interface
• internal implant connection
• ease of use
• ability to cement or screw-retain final prosthesis
• rationalised componentry
• low start-up costs
• affordable cost to patient
• training, education and ongoing support.

Conclusions

Various treatment options are available for both the partial and fully eden-tulous patient. Implant dentistry has had a long history and previously was more an art than a science. Implantology is now an accepted treatment option, with endosseous implants providing a predictable prognosis for the patient. Careful consideration should be given to the factors affecting success, surgical technique and choice of implant.

Further Reading

Brånemark P, Zarb T, Albrektson T. Tissue-Integrated Prostheses. London: Quintessence Books, 1985.

Esposito M, Hirsch JM, Lekholm U, Thomsen P. Biological factors contributing to failures of osseointegrated oral implants. (1) Success criteria and epidemiology. Eur J Oral Sci 1998;106:527-551.

Esposito M, Hirsch JM, Lekholm U, Thomsen P. Biological factors contributing to failures of osseointegrated oral implants. (2) Etiopathogenesis. Eur J Oral Sci 1998;106:721-764.

Chapter 2
Case Selection

Aim

The aim of this chapter is to discuss the reasons for tooth loss and how this may influence the method of replacement. We will examine the need to replace missing teeth and outline the advantages and disadvantages of each method of tooth replacement.

Outcome

After reading this chapter the reader should have an understanding of how the aetiology of tooth loss influences treatment planning and the options available for tooth replacement.

Introduction

Dental implants may be considered the means of tooth replacement of choice in modern dentistry. It should not be forgotten, however, that there are other methods of tooth replacement that should be considered each time the patient asks for a tooth space to be filled.

Reasons for Tooth Loss

The reason for the loss of the teeth must be ascertained, as this can often influence treatment planning. The prognosis of the dentition as a whole, together with the prognosis for the teeth adjacent to the tooth space, must be determined. If further tooth loss is anticipated, then contingencies for subsequent tooth replacement must be built into any treatment plan. In cases in which the prognosis of the remaining dentition is poor a radical treatment plan may prove to be more beneficial to the patient in the long term. Depending on the nature of the dental disease and the ease of tooth extraction there will be a variable degree of soft and hard tissue loss once the teeth have been removed. With implants tissue loss should be minimal, but in severe cases of tissue loss a compromised result may occur unless some form of augmentation is considered.

The main reasons for tooth loss or missing teeth are as follows:
- periodontal disease
- dental caries
- endodontic failure
- trauma
- hypodontia.

Periodontal Disease

If the patient has advanced progressive periodontal disease there should be concern for the prognosis of the whole dentition. The patient in Fig 2-1 displays features of an unstable dentition with a poor appearance. Conventional tooth and implant abutments may be equally at risk from future bone loss. Progression of periodontal disease leads to recession and loss of soft tissues. This results in lengthened clinical crowns and the appearance of "black triangles" interdentally. This will lead to a poor aesthetic outcome unless flanges are considered on bridgework or partial dentures. With dental implants some form of soft tissue or bone augmentation is typically required.

Dental Caries

Dental caries weakens tooth structure. Treatment of dental caries with plastic or cast restorations results in further loss of tooth structure. The restorative cycle of repair and replacement further weakens the tooth so that endodontic treatment may be required, followed by the need for auxiliary retention by means of pins or posts. The potential for early failure of heavily restored teeth makes treatment-planning uncertain.

Endodontic Failure

Endodontic treatment is generally successful. Success rates of 95% over 10 years have been published. However, limited coronal tooth structure is of

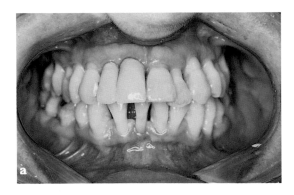

Fig 2-1 (a) An unstable periodontally compromised dentition with impending tooth loss. (b) Orthopantomogram showing severe irregular bone loss.

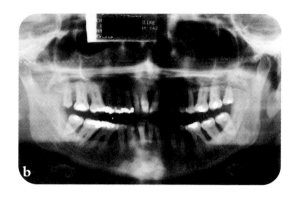

greater concern. The lack of remaining tooth structure leaves the tooth weakened and sometimes necessitates a post and core to retain a crown. Not infrequently the endodontic treatment remains satisfactory, but further loss of tooth structure or root fracture leads to tooth loss (Fig 2-2). When endodontic failure occurs repeat treatments may suffer limitations, in particular if surgical endodontics are required on heavily restored teeth. It is useful to fully assess the expected prognosis of such teeth and to carry out a cost/benefit analysis of retreating them. Often it may be more appropriate to consider removal and replacement of the tooth rather than attempting a repair or replacement restoration.

Trauma

Severe trauma may lead to hard and soft tissue loss. Teeth may be avulsed or fractured. It is often difficult to predict the prognosis of traumatised teeth. A significant proportion of such teeth lose their vitality perhaps five to 10 years after the initial trauma. This reduces their ability to perform as potential abutments for bridges or dentures. Traumatised teeth can be affected by internal and external resorption.

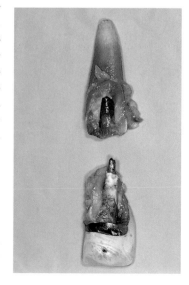

Fig 2-2 Vertical root fracture of a central incisor tooth restored with a post crown, necessitating extraction.

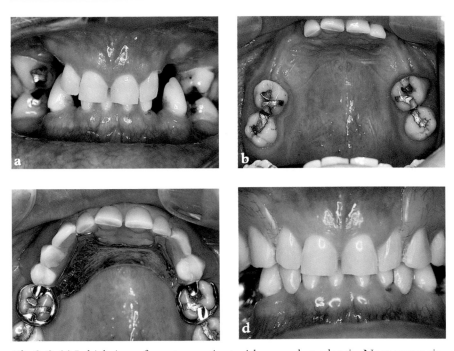

Fig 2-3 (a) Labial view of a mature patient with severe hypodontia. Note severe tissue hypoplasia in the canine and premolar regions (b) Palatal view showing lack of suitable abutments for bridgework (c) Case restored with a metal framework partial denture (d) Labial view of completed case.

Hypodontia

Approximately 6% of the population are affected by hypodontia or congenital absence of teeth. This also includes patients with cleft lip and palate or other craniofacial anomalies. These patients often have microdontia and malocclusions. Where teeth are missing, the alveolar ridge is often narrow or wasted. This complicates orthodontic treatment and subsequent tooth replacement – for example, Fig 2-3 shows a partial denture for a patient with hypodontia. Bridgework was considered inappropriate, and the patient did not wish to consider a bone graft.

Why Replace Missing Teeth?

Patients' expectations of dentistry vary greatly. Most expect to have anterior teeth replaced to restore their appearance. The decision to replace posterior

teeth is often more difficult. Traditionally, the reasons for replacing teeth include:
- appearance
- function
- maintenance of oral health.

Following an extraction, it is not possible to predict whether any adverse tooth movements will occur. There is always the possibility of teeth tilting or drifting into the edentulous space within the same dental arch. Similarly, if the occlusion is unstable the opposing teeth may erupt into the edentulous space. It has been observed that food packing, dental caries, occlusal abnormalities and temporomandibular joint (TMJ) dysfunction, let alone other dental conditions, have ensued following adverse tooth movements. Conversely, it has been shown that, if such tooth movements have not occurred within five years of tooth extraction ,it is very unlikely they will occur in the future. Therefore, if it is decided not to replace lost teeth immediately the situation should be reviewed for periods of up to five years before the edentulous space can be considered stable and left alone with any confidence.

Patients have their own individual smile. This generally includes all the anterior teeth and in some extreme cases the molar teeth. If the smile-line is generous and there is an extensive show of the gingivae, dentists understandably become more concerned about providing a solution to missing teeth.

It is not necessary to have teeth to ingest sufficient food to survive. However, the enjoyment and efficiency of mastication is severely reduced when multiple teeth are missing. It is a subjective decision by the patient as to whether he or she has sufficient teeth to enjoy food. In recent years "shortened dental arch" therapy has gained popularity. It is important to note that the individuals who conceived this concept felt that a reduced number of occlusal units was acceptable as long as patients were not affected by progressive dental disease and, in particular, showed no evidence of TMJ dysfunction, severe tooth wear or periodontal drifting of teeth. Rather confusingly, it remains uncertain as to whether a lack of posterior support leads to such dental conditions. Nevertheless, in masticatory efficiency studies it has been shown that the function of removable partial dentures is grossly inferior to that of the natural dentition, fixed bridgework and implant retained prostheses.

Both the dentist and the patient must be convinced of the need for tooth replacement before treatment options are considered.

Options for Replacing Teeth

Whenever tooth replacement is indicated, the following options should be considered:
- accepting the space
- orthodontics to close the space
- partial denture
- full denture
- overdenture
- conventional bridge
- resin-bonded bridge
- fixed and removable solutions
- dental implants.

The decision to accept the tooth space is usually confined to the posterior regions. The occlusion may be considered stable, but in many cases patients may simply choose to accept the space as they do not perceive a need for tooth replacement.

Orthodontic Treatment

There is obviously great benefit in avoiding any restorative or prosthetic replacement if orthodontic treatment can resolve the problem. Consideration of orthodontic treatment to close spaces is largely limited to younger patients, as adults are less inclined to undergo lengthy treatment involving fixed appliances. Before orthodontic treatment is started to close the space, consideration should be given to the following:
- Technical feasibility -the use of a mock-up will give an indication of the final outcome.
- Oral health – orthodontic treatment is contraindicated in patients with poor oral hygiene.
- Patient commitment – patient's willingness and commitment to undergo lengthy treatment with long-term appliances.
- Stable outcome – following movement teeth need to be stabilised so that a relapse does not occur.

Removable Dentures

Removable dentures have the advantage that they can replace any number of teeth, including the complete dentition. They are the least expensive option to replace teeth and for many patients still remain acceptable. In general, the larger the partial denture becomes the more difficult it is for the patient to manage. When very few, perhaps only two to three teeth remain, consideration should be given to a dental clearance and complete dentures. However, if some roots can be retained, an overdenture may provide an alternative approach. The main advantage for overdentures is that the retained roots are able to preserve alveolar bone, which enhances the success of complete and partial dentures. Depending on the wear of acrylic components and whether the patient is a bruxist or not, acrylic dentures may be expected to last between three to five years before some form of maintenance or replacement is required. A well-made, close-fitting cobalt chrome framework should last in excess of 10 years. However, it is difficult to provide ideal design features and thicknesses of the metal for minor connectors and clasps to last this period of time. Nevertheless, cost is relatively low when compared to fixed replacements. Patients with dentures must be informed of the potential increase in oral disease and their level of homecare commitment to avoid damaging periodontal disease and caries.

Resin-Bonded Bridgework

Since the introduction of adhesive techniques it has been possible to restore many small edentulous spaces with resin-bonded bridges. These can provide a very satisfactory restoration with minimal tooth preparation. Resin-bonded bridgework requires a substantial amount of remaining tooth structure for the restoration to be successful. The longevity of resin-bonded bridges is found to be seven to eight years, with little variation between splinted, cantilever and fixed/fixed designs. This may appear surprising to many practitioners who have limited success with this type of bridgework and view such bridges as technique-sensitive. Considerable care with the laboratory work and metal surface treatment, together with a careful clinical technique, including excellent moisture control, will contribute to successful resin-bonded bridgework (Fig 2-4).

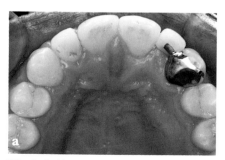 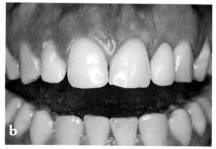

Fig 2-4 (a) Cantilever resin-bonded bridge replacing a lateral incisor tooth in a 14-year-old patient too young to be considered for a dental implant (b) Labial view of resin-bonded bridge.

Resin-bonded bridges are not considered appropriate in the heavily restored dentition where enamel surfaces are sparse.

Conventional Bridges

Conventional bridges were often considered the ideal treatment for the restoration of the partially edentate patient. Good-quality conventional bridgework may be expected to last in excess of 15 to 20 years (Fig 2-5). As the amount of remaining tooth structure diminishes so do success rates with conventional bridgework. Well-known risk factors include periodontal disease, endodontic treatment, post retention and lack of tooth structure. Success rates will further reduce as the span of the bridge increases.

Conventional bridgework may be difficult to maintain, and failures often result in remakes rather than repairs. The most disappointing failures often result in the loss of abutment teeth. Probably the worst failures are the result of over-ambitious treatment-planning with poor execution and inadequate maintenance. When the length of an edentulous span increases and a free-end saddle is created following tooth loss, it may often be best to consider a combination of crowns and a removable partial dentures. The remaining teeth can be modified to enhance the denture design by providing rest seats, guide planes and appropriate undercuts. Alternatively, full crowns with precision attachments or milled shoulders can greatly enhance denture retention and stability.

Dental Implants

One of the main advantages of using dental implants is that they can replace teeth without involving natural tooth abutments. In many circumstances it

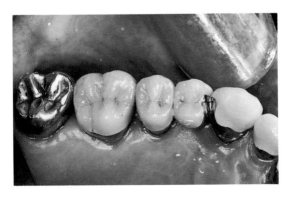

Fig 2-5 A conventional fixed-moveable bridge replacing a premolar tooth in a heavily restored dentition.

may be that heavily restored teeth can be satisfactorily restored with crowns, but they may not be suitable as bridge abutments. Dental implants may be the treatment of choice in the following situations:
• unrestored dentition
• heavily restored dentition (failed bridgework)
• spaced dentition
• lack of suitable abutments (microdont teeth and lack of tooth structure)
• problematic denture wearer (poor anatomy and gag reflex).

Similarly there are circumstances where it is difficult or inappropriate to consider dental implants (that is, where implants may not help your patient):
• poor prognosis dentition
• lack of interdental space (lower anterior teeth)
• lack of interocclusal space
• young patients who have not completed growth.

Conclusions

• The prognosis for individual teeth and the whole dentition needs to be estimated. Teeth with a poor prognosis may be best removed or their future loss anticipated with a 'plan for failure'.
• Soft- or hard-tissue loss will compromise the appearances unless augmentation is considered.
• Not all teeth need to be replaced – some spaces may be accepted and a 'shortened dental arch' may be a reasonable option for some patients.
• Orthodontics can close some spaces. Dentures and bridges should always be considered as alternative prostheses for tooth replacement. Implants are the treatment of choice for most edentulous spaces.

Further Reading

Wise MD. Failure In The Restored Dentition: Management and Treatment. London: Quintessence Publishing Co. Ltd., 1995.

Hemmings K, Harrington Z. Replacement of missing teeth with fixed prosthesis. Dental Update 2004;31:137-147.

Chapter 3
Patient Assessment and Treatment-Planning

Aim

The aim of this chapter is to discuss the importance of obtaining a thorough medical history and clinical patient assessment before embarking on tooth extraction and starting implant therapy. The techniques available to aid patient examination are covered briefly.

Outcome

After reading this chapter the reader should be familiar with the systematic approach used for obtaining a patient history and carrying out a clinical examination.

Introduction

A systematic approach to patient assessment is required. It is carried out in a very similar way to any assessment of a patient needing prosthodontic treatment. The mystique that sometimes surrounds implant therapy should be dispelled. It is worth noting, however, that implant therapy is an unforgiving discipline, and patient expectations are often high.

Clinical Assessment

The first part of the assessment is to define the patient's requirements and expectations. Unrealistic expectations need to be identified and discussed. This is particularly important when significant hard and soft tissue has been lost and when the placement of multiple implants is critical to a successful aesthetic outcome.

Medical History

A full medical history is taken. In addition to the usual contraindications for surgery, it is important to pay particular attention to the following:
• smoking

- uncontrolled diabetes
- facial pain
- psychological problems.

Smoking

Although implants may be placed in patients that smoke, failure rates are considerably higher in smokers, with the probability that the failure rate increases with the extent of smoking. The risks need to be evaluated and carefully explained to the patient. Ideally he or she should be encouraged to stop smoking.

Diabetes

Implants can be placed in patients with diabetes if the condition is controlled. Uncontrolled diabetes should be stabilised before contemplating implant placement.

Facial Pain

The origin of any facial pain needs to be carefully diagnosed, with specialist help as appropriate. Particular care must be taken with patients suffering from "atypical facial pain", as an implant may become a focus for this pain, leading to an intractable problem.

Psychological Problems

The suitability of patients with psychological disorders needs to be assessed most carefully before agreeing to proceed with treatment.

Dental History

A full dental history, including detailed extra- and intraoral examination, is essential. Special attention needs to be paid to progressive periodontal disease, active caries and destructive parafunctional activities.

If split roots, typically relating to post crowns, are present these tend to be associated with rapid bone loss and should be removed as a matter of urgency to preserve a possible implant site.

Clinical Examination

Extraoral

A full extraoral examination should be carried out, with particular attention being paid to the following:

- temporomandibular joints (TMJ) and muscles of mastication
- facial profile and lip support
- smile line.

The TMJ and muscles of mastication are examined for anatomical abnormalities, signs of dysfunction and pathology.

The facial profile and lip support, with and without any existing denture, needs to be carefully evaluated and any atypical features noted.

The smile line relates to the level of the upper and lower lips in relation to the corresponding gingival margins. The smile line is of particular importance in cases in which gingival defects and long teeth are included in the smile. A high lip line may be demanding aesthetically.

Intraoral

A comprehensive intraoral examination must be completed, with special attention to a number of general and site specific features (Fig 3-1) as follows:
- General:
  - primary disease
  - parafunction (Fig 3-2a)
  - prognosis of remaining teeth
  - occlusal support and control.
- Specific to site:
  - space-interdental and interocclusal
  - ridge thickness and shape
  - nature, thickness and condition of the soft tissues
  - availability of bone, taking account of features such as concavities.

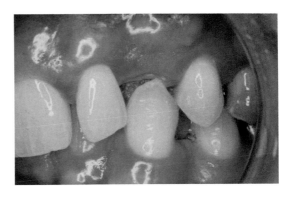

Fig 3-1 Lack of occlusal space.

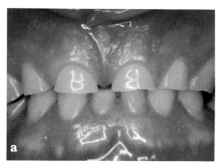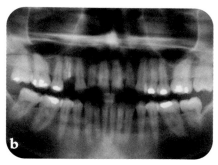

Fig 3-2 (a) Tooth wear caused by parafunctional activity. (b) Axial tomogram used for initial assessment.

Study Casts

It is invariably necessary to obtain articulated study casts to allow a well-considered treatment plan to be formulated.

Radiographic Examination

Radiographic examination is required to evaluate the quantity and, as best as possible, the quality of bone available for implant placement. It is also essential to identify and locate anatomical structures. The radiographs need to be accurate to allow for precise measurements to be made before implant placement. The structures of particular interest include:
• Maxilla:
  – maxillary sinus
  – nasal floor
  – incisive canal
  – labial concavities.
• Mandible:
  – inferior dental canal
  – mental foramen
  – lingual concavities.

The radiographic examinations need to balance accuracy and diagnostic value against the exposure to ionising radiation. The techniques available for radiographic examination include:
• axial tomograms (DPT/OPG)
• long-cone periapical radiographs
• computed tomography (CT) scans

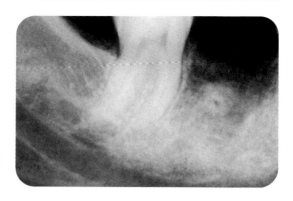

Fig 3-3 Periapical radiograph showing clearly the inferior dental alveolar nerve.

- computer-guided technology
- tomograms.

Axial Tomograms

Axial tomograms give an excellent overall view of the jaws and teeth and are usually the first radiograph taken as part of an implant assessment. The images are enlarged and, as a consequence, it is essential to know the magnification of the machine used. The range is typically x1.2 to x1.4. As panoramic images suffer limitations of accuracy, further radiographs are normally indicated. Any object falling outside the focal trough will not be seen (Fig 3-2b).

Long-Cone Periapical Radiographs

Long-cone periapical radiographs provide an accurate two-dimensional image of anatomical structures. Direct measurements may be made from these images. Periapical radiographs are essential in almost every implant investigation (Fig 3-3).

CT Scans

CT scans give a very accurate view of anatomical structures. Direct measurements can be made from them. The scans provide three-dimensional information in cross-sectional views with indications in assessing both the maxilla and the mandible. In the maxilla, a CT scan is helpful when a large area needs to be investigated. It is especially useful for assessing sinus anatomy and the presence or absence of sinus pathology. In the mandible, a CT scan illustrates lingual concavities and the position of the inferior dental canal. It is not considered necessary to use CT scans routinely when assessing the position of the inferior dental canal. The radiation dose to patients is relatively high and, as a consequence, there must be clinical justification for all scans (Fig 3-4).

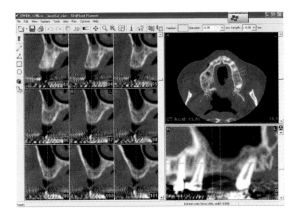

Fig 3-4 CT scan showing sectional views of maxilla.

Computer-Guided Technology (CAD-CAM)

Surgical planning software and computer-guided implantology – for example, SimPlant (Columbia Scientific Inc, Maryland, USA), coDiagnostiX (IVS Solutions, Chemnitz, Germany) and MED3d (med3D GmbH, Heidelberg, Germany) allows for the interactive use of CT data and combines the 3D accuracy of CT imaging with computer-aided design. It enables precise preoperative assessment and treatment planning before implant placement. It is possible to simulate surgery and place virtual implants with geometric accuracy to the nearest millimetre.

If an appropriate radiographic orientation device has been used at the time of scanning, surgical guides can be constructed by CAD-CAM technology. This allows the operator to plan the case, place virtual implants and then construct a surgical guide to aid implant placement. As with CT scans, there is also some ability to make a qualitative assessment of the bone (Fig 3-5).

Tomograms

Tomograms also provide 3D information and cross-sectional views but are limited to short sections of the mandible and maxilla. Tomograms tend to be less accurate than CT scans and may be distorted — in particular if positioning is not optimal. The main use of tomograms is to provide cross-sectional views of limited anatomical sections — for example, in inferior dental canal localisation and in the assessment of lingual concavities. The main advantage of tomograms over CT scans is the reliance on less expensive equipment. However, when large areas are to be investigated and multiple tomogram sections required, CT scans are preferable as exposure to ionising radiation is reduced (Fig 3-6).

It is advisable to use a combination of radiographic views to reduce the chance

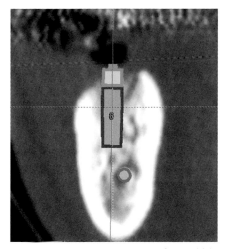 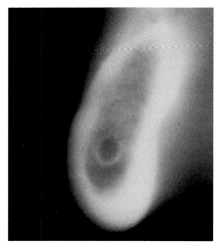

Fig 3-5 CT cross-section of mandible showing virtual implant in position and highlighted inferior dental canal (Sim-Plant).

Fig 3-6 Spiral tomogram (Scanora, Soredex, Orion Corporation, Helsinki, Finnland) of posterior mandible showing inferior dental canal and cortical bone.

of error. The combination of an axial tomogram and periapical radiographs is normally sufficient for the majority of implant procedures (Table 3-1).

Treatment-Planning

Following the detailed examination and discussion of the patient's wishes and expectations, decisions can be made and a treatment plan formulated.

Table 3-1 **Typical effective dose for various radiographic techniques**

Techniques	Dose
Periapical	0.003mSv
Axial tomogram (OPG)	0.004mSv
Spiral tomogram (Scanora)	
Maxilla	0.192mSv [1 section 8mm]
Mandible	0.216mSv [1 section1.6mm]
CT scan	
Maxilla	0.042mSv
Mandible	0.073mSv

*CT values refer to helical CT scanner using 60mA and Dentoscan Software.

All options must be considered and presented to the patient, together with details of the advantages, disadvantages, risks, costs and anticipated success. It is felt by some that implants should be the last resort and teeth should be maintained at all costs. The high success rate of implant therapy questions this opinion.

Once the decision to provide an implant-supported prosthesis has been taken, the case must be planned in detail to span all the necessary stages and the various procedures. Any other approach invariably leads to unnecessary difficulties. An essential part of the planning stage is to ensure that the environment in which the prosthesis is to be placed is as favourable and stable as possible.

Controlling the Environment

Using the study casts and a diagnostic wax-up of the proposed restorations it is possible to predict, with a substantial degree of certainty, the final outcome before starting treatment. A careful note should be made of the following:
• proposed occlusal scheme
• prognosis of the teeth that are key to the success of the treatment
• contingency plans if any of the key teeth are lost.

The requirements of the proposed occlusal scheme are posterior stability and controlled anterior guidance. The aim of posterior stability is to distribute axial loading among a reasonable number of posterior teeth. The aim of controlled anterior guidance is to distribute non-axial loading away from the prosthesis wherever possible. If occlusal loading is not controlled in this way, excess loads may be applied to the implants. Remaining teeth should therefore be adjusted and restored, as indicated clinically, to create the occlusal scheme most favourable to the long-term success of the implant-supported prosthesis.

When an implant-supported prosthesis is placed, allowance must be made for the physiological movement of remaining teeth and the implant being, in effect, ankylosed. This usually means keeping implant prosthesis and teeth separate.

The prognosis of the teeth that are key to the success of the implant prosthesis must be assessed carefully by clinical and radiographic means. Where the prognosis is suspect, steps should be taken to limit long-term uncertainties. For example, it may be appropriate to place cast restorations on "key teeth" that have a significant risk of fracture.

Contingency plans for the possible loss of "key teeth" need to be formulated and recorded before starting treatment. If the loss of a "key tooth" would seriously jeopardise the success of the treatment, and the prognosis of that "key tooth" is poor, its removal and replacement should become part of the treatment plan.

Extraction of Teeth

Whether to extract functional teeth or not when considering implant placement is a difficult decision. The final judgement is influenced by the answers to the following questions:
- What is the prognosis and strategic importance of the remaining teeth?
- Will maintaining a tooth complicate treatment in such a way as to be detrimental to the overall treatment goal?
- Will the failure of a tooth with an uncertain prognosis jeopardise the case and entail extensive correction?
- Would leaving the tooth endanger adjacent implants?
- Would a good implant site become a poor one if the tooth were left in place too long?
- Is the outcome of the implant treatment sufficiently certain to justify the sacrifice of the tooth?

Timing of Extractions

When a tooth is to be extracted and replaced with an implant, it is necessary to decide whether this should happen immediately or following a period of healing before placement of the implant. The period required for soft-tissue healing is about one month. For bone healing it is usually in excess of four months. The benefits and problems relating to these alternative approaches are listed below.

Delayed Placement

Potential benefits:
- Initial remodelling of soft and hard tissues has occurred. This allows for predictable placement of implants in relation to these tissues.
- There is more soft tissue available to modify gingival aesthetics.
- It is easier to place the implant after bone healing.

Potential problems:
- Delay in completion of treatment and, if present, prolonged use of a removable denture.

- If the bone ridge is just wide enough for implant placement at the time of extraction then further resorption may occur if placement is delayed, making subsequent implant placement difficult without tissue augmentation.

Immediate Placement of Implant into Extraction Site

Potential benefits:
- Reduces time between removal of teeth and restoring the implant.
- May preserve bone.

Potential problems:
- It may be difficult to decide on the depth to which to place the head of the implant, as hard and soft tissue remodelling varies as the site heals. This may result in either the implant being placed deeper than is ideal, or in exposure of an implant that has been placed too superficially. Multiple units placed in aesthetic areas are particularly vulnerable to these variations.
- Immediate placement may limit the possibility of surgically modifying the soft tissue, as is sometimes necessary to achieve good aesthetics.
- It is a more difficult procedure.

The Number and the Position of Implants

When formulating a treatment plan involving implants, it is essential to be acutely aware of the dimensions required for implant placement. A minimum of 5mm is required in terms of interocclusal space. The minimum mesiodistal space for the placement of a single tooth implant is approximately 6-7mm. For the replacement of some lower incisors and other such situations thin, narrow implants exist. The strength of such implants, however, may be cause for concern.

The planned number and positioning of implants is determined by the proposed restoration, the quantity and quality of the available bone and the loads to which the restoration will be subjected. Some examples are given below by way of a guide:
- *Full maxillary fixed bridge* - typically six implants may be used, but possibly more when available bone is not ideal, or occlusal loads are expected to be high. The implants should be placed at regular intervals and correspond to the correct tooth position for the proposed restoration. Limited cantilevers may be considered.

- *Full mandibular fixed bridge* — implants are typically placed anterior to the mental foramina and, if required, distal to the formina, but clear of the inferior dental canal. Bone quality in the mandible is normally better than that found in the maxilla. This may create an opportunity to use fewer implants in the mandible than would be required in the maxilla.
- *Partial bridge* — if three or more units are to be restored, and assuming that the units are to be linked, it is desirable to distribute loads by arranging the implants in a tripod relationship to each other. If this is achieved, it is not necessary to place one implant for each missing tooth.
- *Maxillary overdenture* — these are typically supported by four implants. Various attachments, including bars and studs, may be used, assuming good separation between the implants.
- *Mandibular overdentures* — two implants are usually all that is required to retain a mandibular overdenture. If a bar is to be used, the implants should be placed anteriorly so that a straight bar can be provided. This has the additional advantage of the bar not encroaching on the lingual space.

With all overdentures it is essential to have adequate interocclusal space for the attachments. Implants may need to be placed deeper into the bone to obtain the space required. Failure to provide adequate space results in over-contoured prostheses and thin acrylic, which is prone to fracture.

Conclusions

- It is essential that implants are placed only in suitable sites in appropriate patients. All treatment options must be considered.
- Medical and dental contraindications must be fully considered before implant placement and a thorough clinical assessment made.
- The most suitable radiographic procedures must be selected to give the required diagnostic information. This has to take into account an up-to-date evaluation of comparative radiation dose.
- Careful treatment planning using all available techniques, including study casts and mock-up of the final result, is required for a predictable clinical outcome.
- A risk assessment is made of the various treatment options, taking into account the prognosis of all remaining teeth. Extraction of compromised teeth may be required to control these risk factors.

Further Reading

Misch CE. Contemporary Implant Dentistry. New York: Mosby, 1993.

Chapter 4
Surgery

Aim

The aim of this chapter is to discuss the basic planning and procedures for implant therapy.

Outcome

After reading this chapter the reader should be familiar with the precautions and procedures necessary to complete implant surgery to the required precision.

Introduction

To carry out precise and successful implant surgery, a thorough knowledge of surgical anatomy and a clear view of the planned prosthetic outcome is required. The surgical techniques described must be as atraumatic as possible to both hard and soft tissues.

Mandible

The main anatomical considerations when placing implants in the mandible include the:
- inferior dental canal
- mental foramina
- submandibular fossae.

Inferior Dental Canal
The position of the inferior dental canal can be a major limiting factor when placing implants in the posterior mandible, as it may restrict the length of implant used. It is therefore essential to locate the canal accurately to allow optimal length of implant to be placed. To achieve this, high-quality radiographs are a necessary part of the preoperative assessment, and supplementary views may be required during the surgical procedure. Surgical exposure and identification of the mental foramen may be helpful in confirming the position of the canal (Fig 4-1).

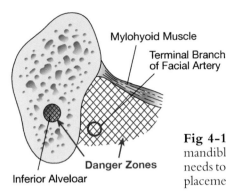

Mylohyoid Muscle

Terminal Branch
of Facial Artery

Danger Zones

Inferior Alveloar

Fig 4-1 Cross-section view of posterior mandible showing where considerable care needs to be taken during surgery for implant placement.

Mental Foramina

The mental foramen defines the site where the inferior dental canal leaves the mandible. Anterior to the mental foramina, it is usually possible to place longer implants, given the amount of bone present. If, however, implants are to be placed close to the foramina, care must be taken that the inferior dental canal has not looped back on itself, leaving a section of the inferior dental nerve anterior to the foramen.

The incisive branch of the inferior dental nerve, which runs anterior to the mental foramen, may be damaged by implants being placed in the anterior mandible. Patients may occasionally comment on some altered sensation in the area. This is usually transient.

Submandibular Fossa

The submandibular fossa is lingually positioned to the body of the mandible below the mylohyoid line. The fossa may limit the placement of implants, especially in the posterior section of the mandible. The anatomical shape of the mandible in the region of the fossa varies considerably and in the posterior region may take the form of a thin lingual shelf through which the unwary may accidentally penetrate. The position of the mylohyoid line can usually be palpated with ease, although it is sometimes necessary to obtain a 3D scan of the area to define the exact shape of the mandible in the region.

The facial artery loops over the submandibular gland in the region of the first permanent molar and gives off a substantial terminal branch in the form of the submental artery. This is at risk of damage in the anterior aspect of the fossa, possibly as far forward as the canine position.

Maxilla

The main anatomical structures to be alert to when placing implants in the maxilla are the maxillary antrum (Fig 4-2) and the incisive canal.

Maxillary Antrum

The maxillary antrum is often a major limiting factor for the use of implants in the posterior maxilla, frequently making implant placement impossible without resorting to bone augmentation procedures. It is worth noting that, if planning to extract maxillary premolar and molar teeth before implant placement, the removal of the teeth may initiate "pneumatisation" of the antrum into the alveolar process. This results in a reduction in the bone available for implant placement.

Incisive Canal

The neurovascular bundle contained within the incisive canal is positioned in the midline, palatal to the central incisor teeth. If implants encroach on this canal, soft-tissue rather than hard-tissue union can be expected in this area. Depending on the extent to which an implant encroaches on the incisive canal, involvement of this anatomical structure may adversely influence the success of the implant placement.

Bone Quality

Bone quality is important in implant success. Typically, the ideal bone is of good vascularity with an adequate cortex and medullary bone of a reasonable density. The anterior mandible is generally considered to be a good site, although penetrating the dense cortex requires a very careful technique to avoid overheating of the bone. The posterior maxilla, which may have eggshell-thin cortex and a sparse medullary space, is generally considered to be the least favourable site for implant placement.

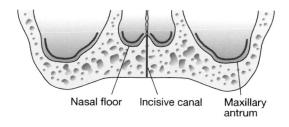

Fig 4-2 Surgical anatomy of maxilla showing sites where implant placement may be restricted.

Nasal floor   Incisive canal   Maxillary antrum

Surgical Technique

The procedure is carried out after careful planning and involves precise soft-tissue handling and bone preparation. The treatment is carried out under sterile conditions. It is essential that bone preparation is made as atraumatic as possible, with heat generation being minimised. Adverse cellular changes can occur within the bone with temperature increases of as little as 4°C. The technique therefore requires intermittent action, controlled operating pressures and copious amounts of saline coolant.

Implant Positioning

The position of implants is dictated by the intended position of the final restoration, not solely by the availability of bone. It must be emphasised that the majority of implant problems stem from lack of adherence to this guiding principle. In particular, care must be taken if different operators carry out the surgical and restorative stages. It is the practitioner who completes the restorative phase, must determine the positioning of implants and communicates this to the surgeon, using a surgical guide if required.

Guidelines for Implant Positioning

The primary guideline for implant positioning is alignment of the implant with the proposed final restoration. Preoperative planning must include consideration of the surgical phase of the treatment.

Preoperative Planning
Radiographs
Presurgical radiographs must be used to assess availability of bone. The use of tomograms and CT scans will provide 3D information (see Chapter 3).

Study Casts
Articulated study casts are invaluable in assessing tooth position, angulation and key features of the edentulous spaces. Measurements can be made and proposed restoration and implant position defined. A diagnostic wax-up on the cast of the proposed restoration can be of great value and will allow the precise construction of a surgical guide. It is important to remember that study casts show soft-tissue shape rather than hard-tissue shape; this may be very misleading. The relationship between bone and soft tissue can be assessed with the aid of radiographs. However, "sounding " the bone and transferring the information to a sectioned cast is a helpful adjunct (Fig 4-3).

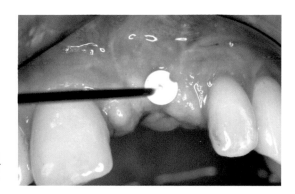

Fig 4-3 Using a straight probe to measure thickness of soft tissue — 'ridge mapping'

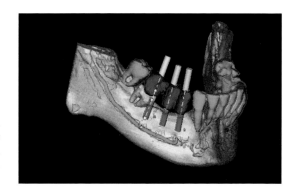

Fig 4-4 CT scan of the mandible using interactive 3D planning and simulated surgery (courtesy of Image Diagnostic Technology Ltd).

Surgical Planning Software
The interactive use of CT data allows for the virtual placement of implants in precise relationship to the proposed final restoration. This surgical simulation allows for 3D planning of treatment before implant placement. The software may also be used to construct computer-generated surgical guides. If this system is used, the accurate location of the guide is essential (see Chapter 3 and Fig 4-4).

Surgical Techniques

The typical relationships and distances between adjacent teeth and implants are shown in Fig 4-5. The typical distance between implants is approximately 3mm. If 4mm diameter implants are used, this translates as 7mm from the centre of one implant to the next. At least 2mm is required between an implant and an adjacent tooth. If implants are placed too close to adjacent

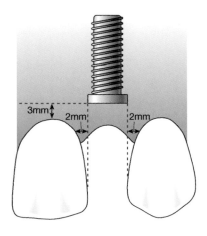

Fig 4-5 The typical relationships and distances between adjacent teeth and implants.

teeth, the intervening bone may be lost, together with the papilla. Surgical guides and location "flags" (for instance, Pallacci flags) can help assist accuracy (Fig 4-6).

The depth to which an implant is placed is critical to the aesthetics and stability of the soft tissues adjacent to the definitive restoration. A significant reference point is the amelocemental junction of the adjacent teeth. The head of the implant should be placed at a depth of 3mm apical to this junction. If placed too superficially, an appropriate emergence profile cannot be produced, and there is a risk of the implant head becoming exposed. If the implant is placed too deeply, the restoration of the implant becomes more difficult and may result in hard- and soft-tissue loss in clinical service.

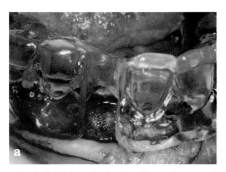
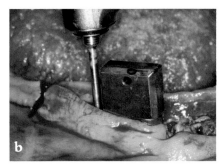

Fig 4-6 (a) Surgical guide in position to define implant location. (b) "location" pallacci flag in position to confirm inter-implant distance.

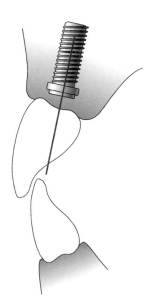

Fig 4-7 Opposing tooth position is a very good guide to implant position. As illustrated, if restoring an upper incisor, the long axis of the implant should approximate with the incisal edge of the lower incisor.

Opposing tooth position is a very good guide to implant position. This is particularly so with screw-retained prostheses. For example, if restoring an upper incisor in a patient with a Class I or II occlusal relationship (Fig 4-7) the long axis of the implant should approximate with the incisal edge of the lower incisor. Notwithstanding the various guidelines that have been described, the clinician may find it necessary to modify implant position at time of placement, depending on soft tissue and bone quality. Such modifications should normally be minor, provided careful planning has preceded the surgery.

First Stage Surgery

Flap Design

This typically involves a full-thickness mucoperiosteal flap, exposing the bone of the proposed implant site and, as necessary, adjacent anatomical structures. Exposure of the site allows the position of adjacent roots to be assessed as well as the bone contour. This is particularly important where bone contour may be unpredictable — for example, the buccal concavity normally present in the apical region of maxillary incisors. The tissues must be handled with care, in particular the interdental papillae. It may be helpful to design the flap to preserve the papillae as shown in Fig 4-8.

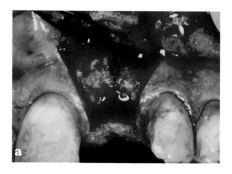

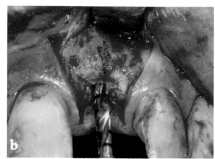

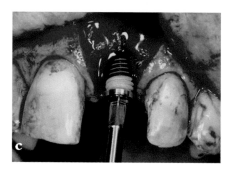

Fig 4-8 (a) Mucoperiosteal flap raised, preserving adjacent papillae and exposing bone contours (b) Preparation for implant using 2mm drill (c) Placement of implant at low speed.

Bone Preparation

Bone preparation is carried out using drills of increasing diameter that gradually widen the site concentrically. Profuse irrigation is essential. The objective is to produce a site as atraumatically as possible into which a slightly wider-sized implant is threaded. The primary goal is to produce rigid fixation of the implant in the bone to ensure its stability during osseointegration. An implant that is not stable at placement is likely to fail and should be immediately removed and either replaced with a wider implant, or the site allowed to heal before making a further attempt at implant placement at a later date. If allowed to fail then bone loss is inevitable. Once in place, a protective attachment (healing abutment) is fitted to the head of the implant.

Single or Two-Stage Surgery

If it is intended to bury the implant during the healing period, a short cover screw or healing abutment is attached. This approach necessitates a second surgical procedure. If a second surgical procedure is to be avoided then a long-healing abutment that protrudes through the soft tissues is fitted. This "single-stage" procedure is not indicated in all situations, in particular, if

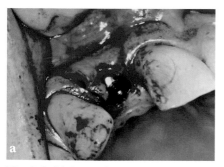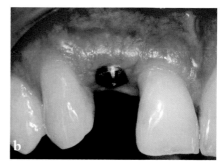

Fig 4-9 (a) Second-stage surgery with flap design to preserve the papillae (b) Site at three weeks post-op.

there is risk of a denture pressing on the integrating implant or, if the implant is short or located in less than ideal bone. If a long-healing abutment is placed, the soft tissue must be carefully adapted around it.

Second-Stage Surgery

Second-stage surgery is required to uncover a buried implant following osteointegration. This may be done using a tissue "punch" or, more typically, by raising a mucoperiosteal flap. The flap is designed to preserve and enhance the soft-tissue profile and contour, with particular attention paid to the interdental papillae. Healing abutments designed to protrude through the soft tissues are attached to the implants during this procedure (Fig 4-9). The impression phase can proceed several weeks later.

Immediate Placement

Immediate placement of implants refers to the placement of the implant into an extraction site immediately following the removal of the tooth. Key aspects of this technique are as follows:

- A basic requirement for implant success is that the implant must be rigidly fixed in bone. As the implant is unlikely to fit an extraction socket perfectly, especially if the implant is of cylindrical design, it is usually necessary to extend the implant apical to the socket to provide this fixation. Immediate implants are rarely placed in molar sites because the position of the inferior dental canal or maxillary sinus usually precludes apical fixation. In addition, the root anatomy of molar teeth tends to make the socket shape unsuitable for immediate implant placement (Fig 4-10).

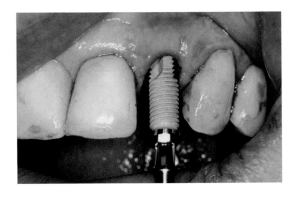

Fig 4-10 Immediate placement of an implant into an extraction socket of 22. No flap has been raised to preserve the papillae - this is only indicated in selected cases.

- The ideal position for an implant is rarely the same as the position of the root socket. This is because allowances need to be made for the bone resorption that follows extraction and the obvious differences between the anatomy of the root and the shape of the implant. Maintaining the socket wall is essential to allow bone, rather that soft tissue, to replace the blood clot that forms between the implant and extraction socket. As the buccal aspect of many tooth roots tend to be covered by very thin bone, great care must be taken during extraction to keep the bony socket intact.
- Immediate implant placement is often technically difficult, as the hard bony socket may influence the direction of implant placement and deflect the implant in an undesirable direction. The technique should be used with caution in aesthetic areas, in particular when multiple teeth are removed and tissue resorption is unpredictable. This may leave the implant unfavourably positioned and inappropriately exposed.

Immediate Loading

Although it is usual to allow implants to integrate before loading, if fixation of the implant is good, the implant may in certain circumstances be loaded immediately. This is a most useful technique in the mandible but may also find application in other areas (Fig 4-11).

Conclusions

- A precise knowledge of surgical anatomy is required before implant placement.
- A careful technique during preparation of the bone is essential to avoid overheating and subsequent damage to the bone.

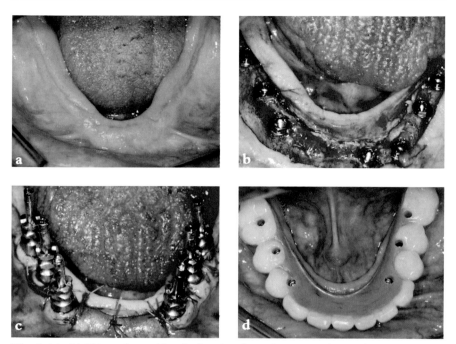

Fig 4-11 (a) Edentulous ridge before implant placement (b) Implants placed (c) Impression copings and abutments in position prior to impression being taken. Great care is taken to contour and close the flap to avoid ingress of impression material. (d) Temporary bridge fitted the following day.

- The exact positioning of the implant in three dimensions is paramount for the ease and success of the prosthetic stages. The use of surgical guides is often recommended.
- Careful manipulation of the soft tissues is required for a good aesthetic result.
- Placement of implants immediately into extraction sockets is a successful procedure if the implant can be rigidly fixed into the bone. This is often not possible for molar teeth given the anatomy of the extraction socket.
- It may be possible to restore implants immediately upon placement; however, in certain situations this may lead to an increased risk of failure.

Further Reading

Palacci P. Esthetic Implant Dentistry: Soft and Hard Tissue Management. London: Quintessence Publishing, 2001.

Chapter 5
Prosthodontic Procedures

Aim

The aim of this chapter is to discuss outline the prosthodontic procedures involved in implant therapy.

Outcome

After reading this chapter the reader should be familiar with the prosthodontic procedures and techniques to be adopted following successful completion of implant surgery.

Introduction

In many ways prosthodontic procedures on dental implants are much simpler than those for conventional crown and bridgework. The ease of restoration depends on the position of the implant. Ideal implant placement is sometimes difficult to achieve, and a functional or aesthetic compromise usually ensues (Fig 5-1). However, the vast majority of implant treatments provide satisfactory functional and aesthetic results. If we are critical of the outcome of implant treatments, the main criticism would relate to the preservation and management of soft tissues, namely the interdental papillae. More often than not when multiple implants are placed there is some reduction of the papillae, referred to as "blunting".

If a machined abutment system is employed, it is relatively easy to achieve an accurate fit of the crown or superstructure. This is in contrast to crown preparation, impression-taking and fitting of conventional crown and bridgework, where it can be difficult to achieve a good fit, in particular if the margins are subgingival. Nevertheless, the prosthodontic procedures involved are broadly similar for the two types of restoration. This chapter will outline the prosthodontic procedures involved following successful completion of implant surgery and the patient presenting with healing abutments in place.

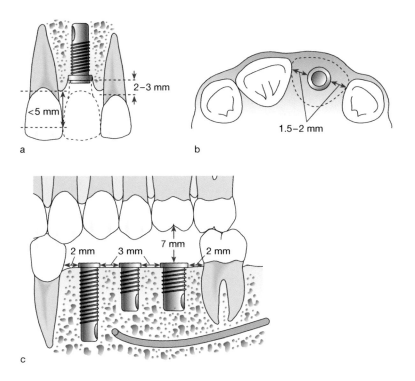

Fig 5-1 (a) Labial and (b) occlusal view of the ideal positioning of a implant for the replacement of an upper central incisor tooth (c) Ideal placement of multiple posterior implants.

Restoration of the Single Tooth Implant

When aesthetics are important, notably in the anterior part of the mouth, the healing abutment should be left in place for approximately five to six weeks following second- stage surgery. This allows the gingival tissues to take up a stable position. When providing posterior restorations, the healing time is not so critical. Some recession of the gingival margin may, however, be anticipated when prosthodontic procedures are started within three to four weeks. The prosthodontic procedures, if machined abutments are used, are as follows:
- removal of healing abutments and placement of machined abutment
- radiographic confirmation of abutment placement
- tightening of the abutment screw with a torque wrench
- impression procedures using an impression coping

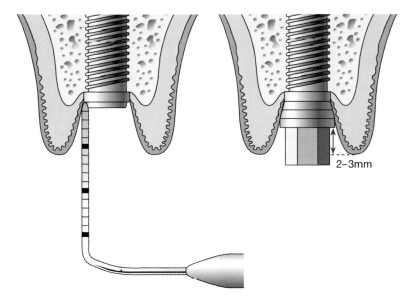

Fig 5-2 Gingival measurement before abutment selection.

- jaw registration
- shade-taking
- temporisation
- try-in and cementation or screw retention.

For anterior teeth, the implant should be aligned in such a way that the long axis is in line with the incisal edges of the adjacent teeth. For posterior crowns, the long axis of the implant should be aligned so that the screw access comes through the central fossa of the premolar or molar tooth. Single-tooth machined abutments are usually provided with a variation in collar height. To optimise the emergence profile of the crown the collar should be 2–3mm below the gingival margin (Fig 5-2). A measuring gauge or a graduated periodontal probe is useful in measuring height from the fixture head to the gingival margin. A surgical stent is also useful at this stage, as an assessment can be made of the screw-access channel relative to the labial face of the tooth. If there is poor positioning of the implant, the use of a customised abutment may be appropriate, as described below.

Torque Wrench
Following radiographic confirmation of correct seating of the abutment to

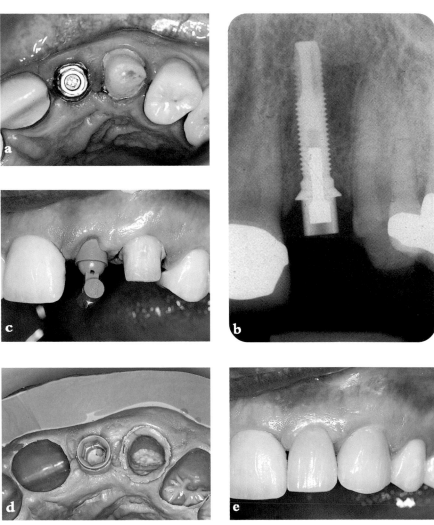

Fig 5-4 (a) Single-tooth abutment to replace an upper lateral incisor tooth. The canine has been an abutment for a temporary cantilever bridge (b) Radiographic confirmation of abutment placement (c) Impression coping in place (d) Impression showing pick-up of impression coping and margins of canine (e) Implant and conventional crown in place.

cedures can be facilitated if a customised abutment is used. With some implant systems angulated abutments are able to overcome certain problems. It is more common, however, for customised abutments to be produced in the laboratory. Impression procedures differ slightly in that a fixture-head impression is required. This means an impression coping is attached directly to the implant fixture head as shown in Fig 5-5. An open-tray technique is required whereby the impression coping can protrude through an opening in the impression tray. After the impression has been taken the impression coping is unscrewed to allow withdrawal of the impression from the mouth. Some implant systems include a "push-fit" attachment for impression copings. In the laboratory, a fixture head–working cast is produced. This allows a customised abutment to be produced, reangulating the retaining core to a favourable position. Such customised abutments can be made of gold alloy, titanium or ceramic. It is good practice to make a temporary crown at this stage. Once the abutment has been placed, a further working impression is required. If the customised abutment and final crown are produced at the same time, small inaccuracies may be included in the final restoration and can detract from the aesthetic outcome. If, however, such inaccuracies can be avoided, the prosthodontic procedure is simplified.

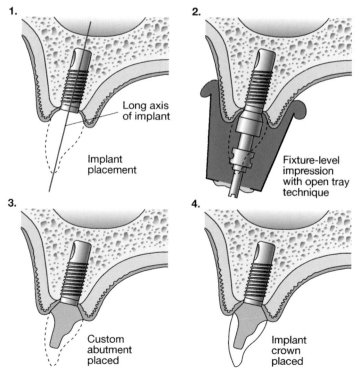

1. Implant placement — Long axis of implant
2. Fixture-level impression with open tray technique
3. Custom abutment placed
4. Implant crown placed

Fig 5-5 Procedure in the prosthodontic phase of implant therapy involving the use of a customised abutment.

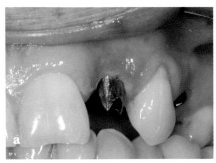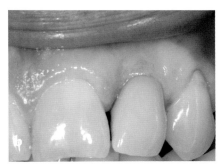

Fig 5-6 (a) Customised abutment in the restoration of a lateral incisor tooth (b) Final restoration.

The success rate of cemented implant crowns appears to be good. Initially there were concerns as to whether cemented crowns and abutments would loosen and there would be some need to employ a retrievable system. Alternatively, single crowns can be made as screw-retained crowns, which incorporate the abutment and attach directly onto the implant, avoiding the need for intermediate abutments. Such crowns may on occasion be more bulky than cemented crowns but are preferred by some clinicians. A single cemented implant crown using a customised abutment is shown in Fig 5-6.

Partial Replacement Case

The complexity of the prosthodontic phase of treatment increases with the number of implants. If screw-retained restorations are planned, the ideal positioning of the dental implants allows the screw access to be lingual to the labial face of the replacement teeth. This is less critical if a cemented bridge is planned, in particular if it involved the use of customised abutments. If the implants are placed deeply, it is possible to use machined angulated abutments to reposition the screw access channels into a more favourable position. If the implants are superficially placed it can be difficult to avoid an exposed metal collar in the completed restoration.

There is a tendency to provide an implant for each tooth to be replaced. This can prove to be highly expensive and to date has no scientific justification. Biomechanical considerations require the application of similar design principles to those employed in conventional bridgework. Higher stresses are generated in prostheses of cantilever design than in prostheses of fixed-fixed designs, in which there is support at each end of the superstructure. However, it is sensible to employ as many implants as possible to distribute loads favourably. Therefore, two dental implants maybe used in the replacement of three teeth, in a form similar to a conventional three-unit fixed bridge, but three implants would individually be subject to smaller loads. The final decision is often influenced by the space available for implants and financial considerations. It should be remembered that 'squeezing' in too many implants may detract from the final appearance.

In partial replacement cases, the prosthodontic procedures are very similar to those for restoring a single tooth implant. As the span increases there are more indications for additional prosthodontic procedures to ensure accuracy of fit and jaw registration. The procedures tend to be as follows:
• abutment selection
• radiographic confirmation of abutment fit and use of torque wrench
• impression procedures
• verification of accuracy of working cast
• jaw registration
• tooth try-in
• metal try-in
• try-in of final restoration placement.

In certain circumstances some of these stages can be undertaken during the same appointment. For example, the use of a Duralay (Reliance Dental Mfg. Co Illinois, USA) bar with copings can verify the accuracy of the working cast and, when placed in the mouth, can be used to facilitate jaw registration procedures. Best accuracy is achieved using pick-up impression copings and an open-tray technique. However, when access is difficult in the posterior regions, it may be easier to use reseated impression copings and a closed-impression tray technique.

Temporisation at this stage may be the patient continuing to wear partial dentures, a temporary conventional bridge or a resin-bonded bridge. Alternatively, a temporary implant bridge can be made. This may be made at the chairside, but tends to be more durable if made in the laboratory. The use of such temporary bridges can allow the clinician to assess the initial aesthetics, the occlusion and the soft-tissue response to the proposed long-term restoration. If the patient has high aesthetic demands, or maintenance of good oral health is difficult, it may be worth spending some weeks or months at this stage before embarking on the very expensive, definitive long-term restoration (Fig 5-7).

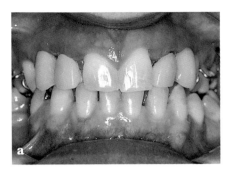

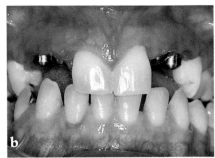

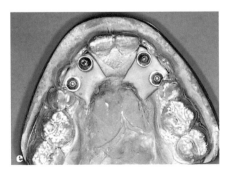

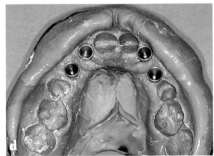

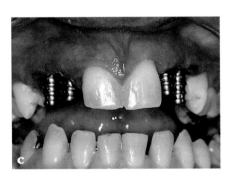

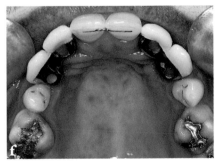

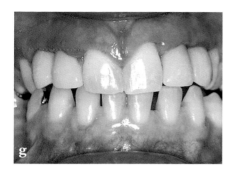
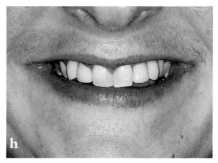

Fig 5-7 (a) Patient with hypodontia restored by means of a partial denture (b) Healing abutments in place (c) Conical impression copings in place (d) Working impression (e) Working cast with surgical template in place (f) Splinted crowns in place. Temporary dressings in screw access holes (g) Labial view of final restorations (h) Smile line showing restorations.

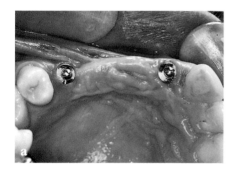
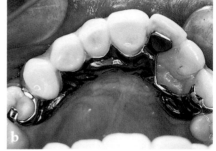

Fig 5-8 (a) Ball-ended attachments (b) Implant overdenture retained by ball attachments.

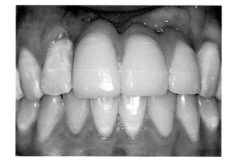

Fig 5-9 Fixed-implant bridge with "pink porcelain" to disguise tissue deficit.

In partial replacement cases, it is usual to provide a fixed bridge restoration. Occasionally, if implant abutments are limited, or there has been a failure during the surgical stage, the use of a removable partial overdenture may be considered as an interim or rescue prosthesis. The construction of an implant-retained removable partial overdenture (Fig 5-8) would follow the same stages as for an edentulous restoration described below.

In many cases, the patient has significant hard and soft tissue loss. If the patient is not willing to consider tissue grafting, or is reluctant to accept the provision of a removable overdenture, the use of an acrylic flange or 'pink porcelain' on a porcelain-fused-to- metal superstructure can produce an acceptable compromise result (Fig 5-9).

Edentulous Case

In the restoration of a complete dental arch by means of implants, two options are available to the practitioner, namely:
- fixed–implant retained bridge
- implant-supported overdenture.

The use of a fixed bridge or overdenture is typically determined by the number of dental implants present and the need for a flange. The following guide may be of assistance in reaching a decision:
- Fixed bridge:
  - maxilla – six implants
  - mandible – four implants
- Overdenture:
  - maxilla – four implants
  - mandible – two implants.

Traditionally, implants were placed only in the anterior part of the mouth where bone was available. With improvements in bone augmentation techniques, it is now more common for consideration to be given to bone grafts to the posterior maxilla and mandible to allow additional implants to be placed. The more implants placed, the greater the chance of providing a fixed-bridge restoration. A mandibular fixed bridge based on four dental implants is shown in Fig 5-10. Such restorations are extremely successful, with the prospect of clinical service in excess of 30 years. The superstucture requires maintenance or replacement on a five- to 10-year cycle, depending on the materials used and the occlusal loads involved. A full arch bridge with good implant support is shown in Fig 5-11. The need for a flange was the

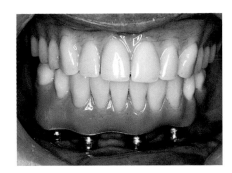

Fig 5-10 Fixed mandibular implant-retained bridge.

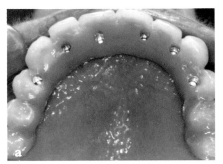

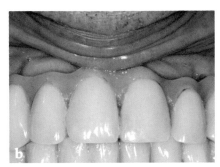

Fig 5-11 (a) Occlusal view of a full arch reconstruction (b) Facial view of full arch reconstruction.

result of alveolar resorption, but the appearance was acceptable to the patient. The prosthodontic stages for a full arch restoration are as follows:
• primary impressions for a special tray
• secondary impressions with an open-tray technique and impression copings
• verification of the cast if multiple implants are used
• jaw registration, which is most likely to require an occlusal rim
• wax try-in
• metal try-in for framework or gold bar for overdenture. A repeat jaw registration can be carried out at this stage
• wax and metal try-in or metal/porcelain try-in
• finish.

With a complete arch restoration much of the planning of tooth position equates to standard prosthetic techniques for complete dentures. Assessment of the occlusal vertical dimension, occlusal plane, tooth position, centre-line, smile-line and retruded contact position (RCP) are all important to the success of the case.

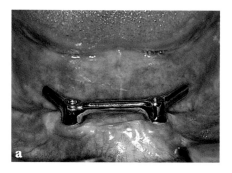

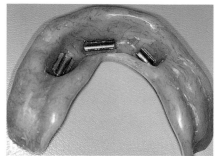

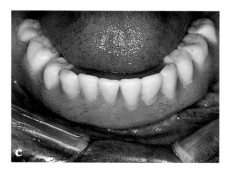

Fig 5-12 (a) Gold bar for implant overdenture (b) Gold clips inserted in implant overdenture (c) Implant overdenture positioned in the mouth.

More often than not there will have been some alveolar resorption. In some cases this can be extreme. To provide a good appearance, including adequate lip support, consideration should be given to the inclusion of a flange in an overdenture or pink porcelain equivalent in a fixed bridge.

Overdentures are often the most cost-effective way of replacing a full arch of teeth using implants. Fewer dental implants are required, as the removable superstructure is partly supported by the mucosa. Such overdentures can be retained in the following way:

- bar and clip
- ball attachments
- magnets.

A bar-and-clip design is the most popular, as it gives the patient confidence with minimal maintenance (Fig 5-12). Ball attachments are simple and allow the patient to clean effectively. It is suggested that ball abutments be used in the mandible and not in the maxilla, given the reported high failure rate for ball attachments in the maxilla. Magnets have certain advantages, but are less commonly used, as they are bulky in design and may corrode in clinical service.

Laboratory Considerations

The success of any prosthodontic treatment is a team effort and depends on many factors, namely:
• patient selection and assessment
• presurgical planning
• implant placement
• prosthodontic procedures
• technical and laboratory support.

The clinician's responsibility is to provide work of the highest possible quality. This should be mirrored in the dental laboratory with accurate and skilled manipulation of materials. Communication and a good relationship between clinician and dental technician reduce the chance of errors. Ultimately, the responsibility for the finished prosthesis lies with the clinician.

For details of laboratory procedures the reader is referred to laboratory manuals produced by each implant company. Preformed or machined copings on to which metal, acrylic, porcelain or composite materials are added facilitate accuracy of fit. The laboratory stages will be familiar to most readers as:
• production of a working cast
• selection of components and design
• wax-up to full contour
• casting of metal superstructure
• veneering with porcelain, acrylic or composite.

Dental materials are constantly evolving to enhance clinical performance and appearance. All-porcelain restorations have been introduced for single-tooth restorations. A strengthened core is cast or milled to fit the fixture head or implant abutment. Surface porcelains are then fired to produce the desired contour and shade.

CAD-CAM

Computer-aided design-computer-aided manufacture (CAD-CAM) has recently been developed for use in implantology. Various procedures have been employed utilising laser scanning, sparked erosion and milling techniques. In this way a single abutment (Figs 5-13) or frameworks can be produced (Fig 5-14).

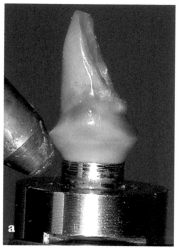 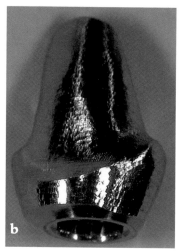

Fig 5-13 (a) Procera scanner scanning a waxed-up coping (b) Computer display of wax coping (c) Milled titanium coping.

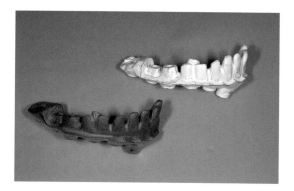

Fig 5-14 Full arch titanium framework.

Key Points

- Prosthodontic procedures have been described for the restoration of single tooth, partial replacement and edentulous implant cases.
- Ideal surgical implant placement allows the use of standard components and impression procedures.
- Fixture level impressions and the use of custom abutments, as is standard practice with some implant systems, allow restoration of difficult cases.

- Cemented implant crowns and superstructures give the best appearance occlusally, whereas screw-retained prosthesis allow easier maintenance.
- Temporary prostheses give the clinician and the patient the opportunity to assess the appearance and function prior to completing the laboratory prescription.

Further reading

Laboratory and clinical procedure manuals for implant treatment - these are produced by each implant company.

Chapter 6
Advanced Cases

Aim

The aim of this chapter is to discuss issues in the management of cases that require advanced implant treatment.

Outcome

After reading this chapter the reader should have insight into the many varied complexities of using implants in more complicated cases.

Introduction

Good implant therapy results should be expected when a single tooth or a small number of teeth that have been removed atraumatically are to be replaced. The prosthetic management conforms to the existing dentition and supportive tissues.

Full Mouth Reconstruction

As the number of teeth to be replaced increases so does the complexity of planning and the provision of treatment. The time required is not proportional to the number of units to be replaced. More time will be required in more extensive cases for both the clinical and laboratory stages. If the dental arch is edentulous, multiple fixtures will be required. It may be that a number of teeth can be saved. In such cases a decision has to be made as to whether to link the implants to the teeth or to provide a number of independent implant retained units.

Aesthetics

It is simpler to achieve a good aesthetic result if a full arch superstructure is wholly implant-supported. The most predictable way of achieving a good aesthetic result in such situations is by means of an implant-retained overdenture. There is good opportunity to control the aesthetics at the wax try-in stage of treatment. The clinician and the technician have full control over the position and arrangement of the teeth, together with the gingival margins and contours of the prosthetic soft tissues. If there has been limited alveolar resorption, there will be problems accommodating the bulk of an overdenture.

When implant-retained fixed bridges are provided, there is less room for manœuvre, as the fixtures dictate the shape of the superstructure. If there has been minimal alveolar resorption, it can be difficult to create ideal gingival contours and emergence profiles, unless the implants have been placed in an ideal position. With further alveolar resorption, pink porcelain is required to simulate gingival tissues. Some fluting of the periphery of the superstructure is important to allow effective cleaning of the implants and mucosa.

When teeth and implants are used to support a superstructure, it becomes particularly difficult to provide a continuous gingival margin and uniform emergence profile for the teeth included in the prosthesis. If very few teeth remain, and they have a dubious prognosis, a case can be made for their removal to simplify implant treatment, improve the aesthetic outcome and enhance long-term success.

Temporary Superstructure

The use of temporary superstructures in full arch cases can be of considerable assistance in developing an acceptable aesthetic outcome. As it is difficult to make durable all acrylic temporary superstructures, their period of placement should be limited to a period of weeks. If the time required for refining the temporary superstructures needs to be longer than this, it is prudent to consider some form of metal or glass fibre-reinforced temporary superstructure. Such superstructures involve more laboratory work and higher costs, but are sometimes essential.

Impression Procedures

Impression procedures are complicated if prepared teeth and implants are included in a single impression. Often multiple impression procedures are required, involving the use of impression copings or, in some cases, Duralay acrylic bonnets on teeth. The aim of a pick-up impression is to locate dies of teeth and implant analogues within a single master working impression from which a master working cast can be produced. It is prudent, and good practice, to verify the accuracy of a working cast. This will reduce the risk of errors in fit and occlusion at later stages. Verification bars to link implant abutments can be made on the working cast, which can then be checked in the mouth. In some circumstances a verification bite fork can serve the same purpose. These are important measures to avoid errors being compounded during the laboratory phase of treatment.

In the past it was difficult to provide large gold–alloy castings of appropriate accuracy for implant superstructures. Casting difficulties are reduced if small units are planned. Various soldering and laser-welding techniques have been developed to join small castings to form large full-arch units, and casting techniques have also improved to accommodate the fine tolerances required. More recently, titanium-milled castings have provided good fit when used with a fixture-head impression technique.

Maintenance of a full mouth reconstruction is simplified if small units have been employed. A porcelain fracture in a three-unit component is much easier to deal with than the same fracture in a 12-14-unit full arch reconstruction. Back-up dentures or temporary fixed bridges are always useful when the replacement or maintenance of such superstructures is required. It therefore follows that the construction and maintenance of a full arch reconstruction, using two fixtures in the mandible and an implant-retained overdenture, is simpler than a full arch fixed bridge supported by eight to 10 implants.

Traditional teaching has advocated avoiding the joining of implants and natural teeth. It is known that teeth have some 3D physiological mobility, but implants have none. It had been thought that joining implants to teeth might result in the early failure of implant screws or the cement lute. Joining implants to teeth can, however, be successful. Gold copings on implants and teeth followed by a cemented superstructure has been found to be a successful approach. A stress-broken design using a fixed-movable joint has also been employed successfully. Another combination is to use conventional cementation of the retainer on the tooth and screw retention only on the implant. It is not known which arrangement will perform best in the long term, but clinical experiences indicate that these combinations are not as problematic as first thought.

Dental Implants and Periodontal Disease

There are two main problems when considering the placement of dental implants in patients who have or have had periodontal disease:

- There is an uncertain prognosis for the remaining teeth.
- There are concerns that a persistent pathogenic periodontal bacterial flora may adversely affect some dental implants, leading to a loss of osseointegration.

In common with all sound treatment planning, primary dental treatment needs should be met before definitive treatment is carried out. In a patient who has severe periodontal disease, with many teeth having a poor prognosis, it is not unreasonable to consider a dental clearance followed by implant therapy. This is a more predictable treatment option than alternatives involving partial dentures or splinted crown and bridgework. It is considered indefensible to place dental implants in a patient who has advanced uncontrolled periodontal disease. There are, however, a number of case reports showing the successful placement of dental implants in patients who have been successfully treated for periodontal disease. While these early results look promising, there is no long-term data.

Severe periodontal disease increases the mobility of natural teeth and is associated with increased recession of the soft tissues and, in many cases, drifting of the teeth. Such presenting features make it very difficult to achieve a good aesthetic result. By way of example, a maxillary implant-retained overdenture, used to replace missing teeth and alveolus, is illustrated in Fig 6-1. The lower arch is stable from a periodontal viewpoint.

Immediate Implant Placement

All extractions of teeth are accompanied by some alveolar resorption and gingival recession. This is accelerated if a mucosal-borne denture is used to replace the lost teeth. Alveolar resorption may be greatly reduced if tooth roots are retained as overdenture abutments. Similarly, if dental implants are

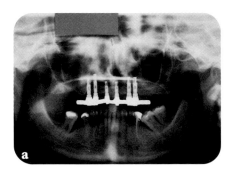 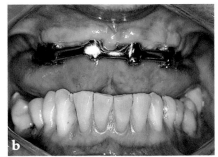

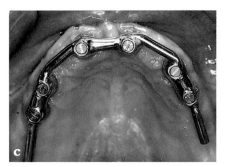
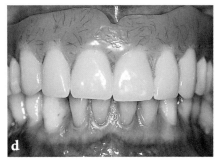

Fig 6-1 (a) Orthopantomogram showing maxillary implant superstructure and bone loss in periodontally stabilised lower arch (b) Facial view and (c) occlusal view of maxillary superstructure (d) Facial view of maxillary-retained overdenture.

placed into an extraction socket, alveolar resorption may be reduced. Immediate implant replacement is worthy of consideration when single-rooted tooth extractions are planned (see Chapter 3). Primary stability of the implants can be achieved if the implant site preparation is deeper and wider than the tooth socket. The use of conical root-form implants may be considered an advantage. If the labial alveolar plate is lost during a difficult extraction, primary implant stability will be difficult to achieve. There are numerous descriptions of using autogenous bone or bone substitutes to fill dead space in extraction sockets as part of immediate implant placement procedures. The use of such materials may not be necessary if a small space exists between the implant and the wall of the socket (Fig 6-2). The technique is generally contraindicated if there is any bony pathology, such as a periapical lesion or following a vertical root fracture. It is also difficult to apply the technique in the sites of multirooted tooth extractions. In such situations, it is preferable to allow healing over three to four months before placement of an implant.

Tissue Augmentation

Substantial loss of hard and soft tissue may occur with trauma, periodontal disease and the treatment of neoplastic disease. In patients with hypodontia the alveolar ridges are underdeveloped, given the absence of permanent teeth. In cases in which the tissue loss occurred some months or years previously, a number of techniques may be used to augment the tissues, namely:
• bone graft
• soft-tissue graft
• guided tissue regeneration (GTR).

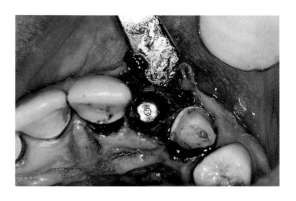

Fig 6-2 Implant placed immediately into an upper lateral incisor tooth socket removed for a root fracture.

Bone Graft

The gold standard for augmentation technique is the use of the patient's own bone. Small amounts of bone can be gathered intraorally from the chin or retromolar areas. If an edentulous area exists this can also be investigated as a donor site. For more extensive bone-grafting/donor sites outside the mouth, such as the hip or ribs, need to be considered. A number of novel techniques have involved harvesting bone from the lower leg and the skull. All these techniques involve a certain amount of morbidity, and much scientific research over recent years has been aimed at providing bone substitutes to reduce risks to patients. Commonly, this has involved the use of sterile hard and soft-tissue substitutes, such as bio-oss (bovine), or inert mineral materials, such as coral or hydroxyapatite. In cases of severe bone loss, corticocancellous bone blocks are required from the hip or ribs to restore whole arches in the form of onlay or inlay bone grafts. These are most commonly placed over the maxilla or into the maxillary sinuses or nasal apertures (Fig 6-3). Usually, large bone grafts are supplemented by packing particulate bone or bone substitutes into the recipient site to create smooth contours. A careful, meticulously planned technique is essential to avoid postoperative complications. In the anterior mandible there is usually sufficient bone to place implants, even in the presence of severe resorption. In the posterior mandible, the inferior dental nerve can preclude simple implant placement. It is often preferable to consider nerve-repositioning or lateralisation of the inferior dental nerve in preference to extensive bone-grafting in this area. This is often associated with some altered sensation, which can be permanent.

Soft-Tissue Grafting

Connective tissue grafts are able to improve gingival or mucosal contours.

They do not, of course, contribute to bone volume, which does not facilitate implant placement if the bone is sparse. They may, however, be used as a supplementary measure if severe tissue loss has occurred. A number of periodontal plastic-surgical techniques exist to regenerate lost interdental or inter-implant papillae. Technique sensitivity exists in this field. The more predictable results rely on a good underlying bone anatomy.

Guided Tissue Regeneration (GTR)

Guided tissue regeneration has been used in periodontal treatment for many years. Its use in implantology is more recent. The same principle of bone healing applies (Fig 6-4) whereby epithelial and connective tissues are excluded from the healing site and bone allowed to grow preferentially

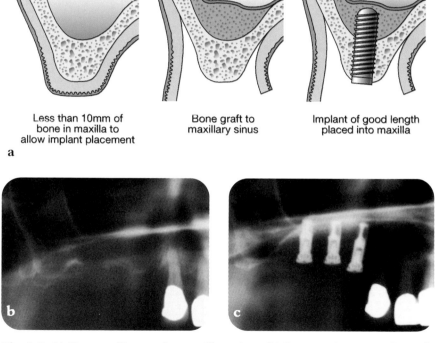

Less than 10mm of bone in maxilla to allow implant placement

Bone graft to maxillary sinus

Implant of good length placed into maxilla

a

b

c

Fig 6-3 (a) Bone grafting to the maxillary sinus (b) Preoperative view of maxilla showing insufficient bone for implant placement (c) Postoperative view showing bone graft followed by implant placement.

around the implant. It is important for the membrane to cover the whole defect and to be held rigidly in place. It is common to use particulate autogenous bone or bone substitutes as part of GTR techniques to enhance bone healing. Bone tacks are usually used to secure the membrane. A novel technique by Simion et al. (2001) involves placing an implant incompletely within the alveolar bone in compromised sites. A guided tissue regeneration membrane is tented over the implant and the dead space filled with autogenous bone or a combination of bone and bone substitutes. This allows bone to grow over the exposed implant surface.

There is no doubt that augmentation techniques can facilitate implant placement and subsequent aesthetics. They significantly increase treatment times, the complexity of treatment and costs. In many clinical situations, however, such techniques may be the only way to allow implant treatment to proceed.

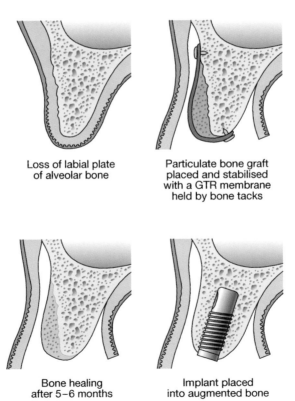

Loss of labial plate
of alveolar bone

Particulate bone graft
placed and stabilised
with a GTR membrane
held by bone tacks

Bone healing
after 5–6 months

Implant placed
into augmented bone

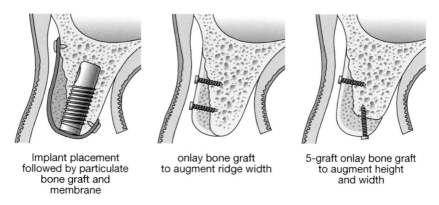

Implant placement followed by particulate bone graft and membrane

onlay bone graft to augment ridge width

5-graft onlay bone graft to augment height and width

Fig 6-4 Bone augmentation using guided tissue regeneration

This is an exciting area of implant research that has resulted in clinical benefits in a relatively short period of time. The use of growth factors or tissue engineering involving scaffold materials and patients' own cells are areas of current research, all aimed at reducing patient morbidity and enhancing success in compromised implant sites.

Immediate Loading

Patients and dentists would like to see the healing times required for implant treatment reduced to a minimum. This has occurred over the past 10 years, and at the time of writing it is considered reasonable to load implants in the mandible three months after placement and five to six months after placement in the maxilla. Many patients would like to have "same-day teeth". This is considered most successful in the mandible (an example is shown in Chapter 4, Fig 4-11). The "Branëmark Novum technique" involves three large dental implants placed using a paralleling technique. A number of precision-engineered parts are required to construct a superstructure onto which prosthetic teeth and flanges can be added. At the time of writing, a small number of centres offer this treatment, but it is technically demanding.

For single teeth or small-span bridges it may also be possible to consider immediate loading. Once implants have been surgically placed, appropriate abutments can be placed on the fixtures as long as they have good stabilisation. This stabilisation can be measured by means of resonance-frequency measurements. While the surgical field is still open, temporary crowns or bridges can be made and cemented or screwed onto the abutments. Thereafter, the soft tissues can be replaced with a careful suturing technique. It is important that the temporary crown or bridge is relieved partially or totally from occlusion in the intercuspal position and lateral excursions (Fig 6-5). Larger-span techniques have been developed to provide temporary implants placed between permanent implant fixtures. Temporary superstructures can be built on these temporary implants for the period of osseointegration, which may be between three to six months, depending on the site in the jaws. The clinician and the patient will incur extra costs with this technique.

Maxillofacial Prosthodontics

The advent of successful implant treatment has revolutionised the results restorative dentists and maxillofacial technicians are able to achieve in patients unfortunate enough to require maxillofacial prosthodontics. In many cases, the severe loss of tissue precludes a successful result with conventional prosthodontic techniques. Patients often have altered sensation and motor function, making it difficult to control removable dentures. The

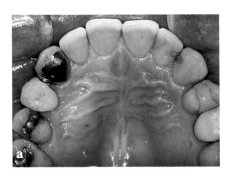
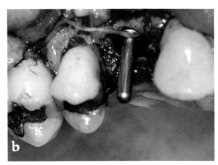
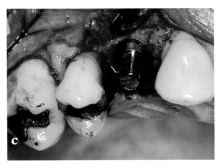
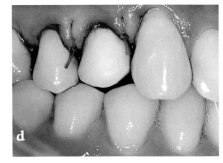

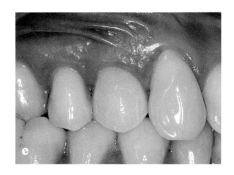

Fig 6-5 (a) Upper premolar temporarily replaced with a resin-bonded bridge (b) Direction indicator showing good position of implant site (c) Implant and abutment placed (d) Temporary crown in place and out of occlusion (e) Final restoration.

denture bearing tissues often have a reduced tolerance, in particular, if they have been subjected to radiotherapy. Xerostomia further complicates the situation and often leads to primary dental disease, if teeth have been preserved. Surgical resection may preclude ideal implant placement. Also, it is recognised that radiotherapy and chemotherapy can lead to delayed healing and reduced implant success rates. Prophylactic antibiotics and hyperbaric oxygen have been used in an attempt to improve implant success rates in affected patients.

For intraoral prostheses, it may only be possible to place a few dental implants, in particular, if there is limited access. A successful result can often be obtained, however, by using an overdenture retained by a bar and clip. If multiple implants can be placed, the possibility of using a fixed bridge remains.

Perhaps the most dramatic improvements achieved in the field have occurred when replacing missing extraoral tissue. Eye, ear and nose prostheses had hitherto been retained by theatrical glue or natural undercuts on the remaining face. Sometimes these prostheses were attached to spectacle frames, if the nose and ears were still present. Short, wide diameter implants can be placed in the relatively thin bones comprising the facial skeleton. The use of bars and clips, studs or magnets has enabled quite large prostheses to be successfully worn by patients (Fig 6-6). The use of implants has also allowed the provision of bone-anchored hearing aids (BAHAs). It is also interesting to note that dental implants have been used to retain other parts of the body, including fingers and other limb extremities.

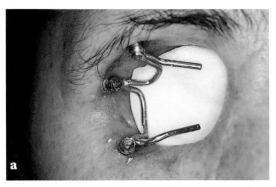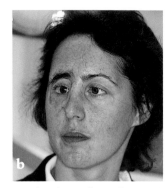

Fig 6-6 (a) Cast framework used to support and retain an orbital prosthesis (b) Facial view of orbital prosthesis.

Conclusions

- Careful planning and extra prosthetic stages are required to ensure accuracy and successful management of the complex case. Implants should not be used in patients with active periodontal disease and with caution in treated periodontal patients.
- Tissue loss will compromise the aesthetic result, but this may be acceptable to patients. Augmentation with hard or soft tissue will facilitate implant treatment and usually improve the appearance.
- Immediate loading is possible in the mandible but is associated with greater risk of failure elsewhere in the mouth.
- Dental implants can stabilise maxillofacial prostheses. Liaison with all health care professionals involved in the care of these patients will increase success rates.

Reference

Simion M, Jovanovic SA, Tinti C, Benefenati SP. Long-term evaluation of osseointegrated implants inserted at time or after vertical ridge augmentation. A retrospective study of 123 implants with one- to five-year follow-up. Clin Oral Implants Res 2001; 12:1, 35-45.

Further Reading

Misch, CE. Contemporary Implant Dentistry. New York: Mosby, 1999.

Bone augmentation for implant placement: keys to bone grafting (chapter 29, pages 451–467)

The maxillary sinus lift and sinus-graft surgery (chapter 30, pages 469–495)

Intraoral autogenous donor bone grafts for implant dentistry (chapter 31, page 497–508).

Whorle. P. Single-tooth replacement in the aesthetic zone with immediate provi-sionalization: 14 consecutive case reports. Pract Periodont Aesthet Dent 1998:10:1107–1114.

Chapter 7
Complications and Maintenance

Aim

The aim of this chapter is to discuss common complications in treatments involving the use of implants and to consider arrangements for the monitoring and maintenance of completed implant cases.

Outcome

After reading this chapter the reader should be familiar with the nature and management of common complications in treatments involving the use of implants. In addition, the reader should be familiar with arrangements for the monitoring and maintenance of completed implant cases.

Introduction

Complications may occur in both the surgical and prosthodontic phases of implant therapy. It is essential to warn patients of the possibility of surgical and postoperative problems. Failure of osseointegration is relatively rare in well-planned cases, with most failures occurring soon after surgical placement or before loading.

Complications in most cases are avoidable by careful attention to diagnosis, treatment planning and good surgical and prosthodontic planning, and by following established protocols of individual implant systems.

Surgical Complications

The more common, relatively minor complications following surgery include swelling, bruising and discomfort. All patients should be warned of these complications and the anticipated extent of them before surgery is undertaken.

As with all minor surgical procedures, surgical complications can be minimised by adequate anaesthesia, gentle surgical manipulation of both hard and

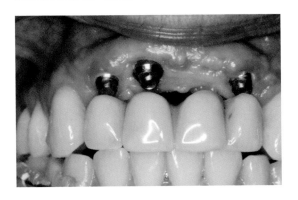

Fig 7-1 Clinical view of an upper partial case displaying poor positioning of the implants in relation to the final tooth position.

soft tissues, pre- and postoperative analgesia, and careful postoperative wound management, including the use of pressure and ice packs to reduce swelling.

Haemorrhage may occur at the time of surgery if there is excessive trauma to soft tissue or damage to aberrant vessels within the bony cortex. Failure to establish good primary stability at the time of implant placement may result in early failure.

Incorrect positioning of implants at the time of surgery, as a consequence of poor planning or lack of necessary skills, knowledge and understanding may result in considerable difficulties during the restorative phase of treatment. It is essential to use surgical guides and templates if positioning problems are to be minimised (Fig 7-1).

Postoperative Pain

Mild postoperative pain is to be expected. It should, however, be readily controlled by means of non-prescription analgesics.

Severe pain following implant surgery is extremely rare. Patients with pain after 24 hours should be monitored for signs of infection, bleeding and other complications. In such situations there may well be an increased risk of implant failure.

The routine use of antibiotics pre- and postoperatively will decrease the possibility of infection. The practitioner must, however, be satisfied as to the indications to prescribe prophylactic antibiotics.

Wound Dehiscence

In the two-stage surgical technique, breakdown of the soft tissue following

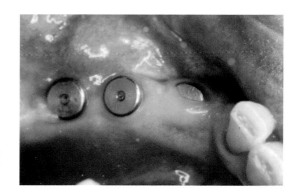

Fig 7-2 Wound dehiscence and exposure of cover screws.

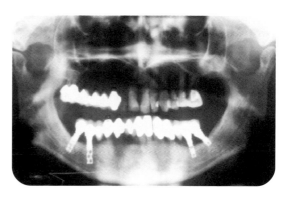

Fig 7-3 A dental panoramic radiograph showing implant on lower right quadrant, which has been placed through the inferior dental nerve, resulting in paraesthesia.

implant placement may lead to the exposure of the implant and cover screw (Fig 7-2). This may be the result of poor soft-tissue coverage of the implant or trauma from the prosthesis covering the surgical site. The diagnosis of the cause of soft-tissue breakdown needs to be established when planning further management of the case. In all cases the surgical sites must be kept clean with antiseptic mouthrinses, such as chlorhexidine, used as indicated clinically.

Paraesthesia
Paraesthesia may arise following trauma to nerves in the region of the implant site. The trauma may be direct from drilling through, or at least into a structure, or indirect as a result of excess heat generation. Whatever the cause, trauma to sensory nerves may lead to loss of sensation to the lower lip (Fig 7-3).

Transient loss of sensation in the lower lip may occur from bruising and swelling of soft tissue around the mental foramina.

Permanent loss of sensation may be the result of damage to the inferior dental nerve. This should be avoided through careful radiographic assessment and including a safer margin for possible error in the planning of implant placement.

Damage to the incisive branch of the inferior dental nerve may result in patients complaining of parasthesia or anaesthesia to any remaining lower incisors.

Mandibular Fractures
In severely resorbed mandibles multiple implants may weaken the jaw with a resultant fracture. This is, however, very rare in suitably planned cases.

Complications Following Second-Stage Surgery

Second-stage surgery involves uncovering of the implant, removal of the cover screw, replacing it with a healing abutment and careful suturing of the soft tissues around the abutment. A careful and gentle surgical technique is essential in minimising complications, notably poor, unaesthetic gingival contour.

Failure to Integrate
Mobility of an exposed implant is indicative of failure of the implant to integrate. The implant and any associated soft tissue should be removed. Immediate placement of a larger diameter implant may be considered. It may be prudent, however, to leave the site to heal, with time to replan treatment.

Excessive Bone over the Cover Screw
Occasionally the cover screw can be partially covered by bone. This bone

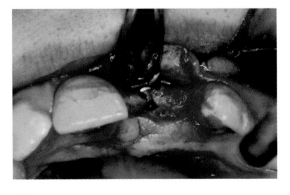

Fig 7-4 Growth of bone over a cover screw, as seen at the time of second-stage surgery.

needs to be cleared away before attempting to remove the cover screw. Most implant systems supply a bone mill for this procedure (Fig 7-4).

Bone Growth between the Cover Screw and Implant
If the cover screw has not been placed directly onto the implant head at the time of first-stage surgery, bone may grow into any gap left between implant head and cover screws. Implant systems include a bone mill for the careful removal of bone from the implant head and thereby provide a clear path of insertion for the abutment.

Prosthetic Complications

Implant prosthodontics can be relatively uncomplicated when fixture angulation and positioning is ideal. In most cases, complications can be avoided by means of careful preoperative treatment-planning and meticulous attention to detail, both clinically and in the laboratory.

Biomechanical Problems

Biomechanical problems may include:
- fracturing of the prosthesis
- loosening or fracturing of abutment screws
- loosening or fracturing of gold screws
- lute failure in a cement-retained prosthesis
- fracture or loss of the implant.

Fracture of the Prosthesis
Fracture of a fixed implant superstructure is often the result of misjudged space, leading to thin sections of materials, errors in technical procedures or

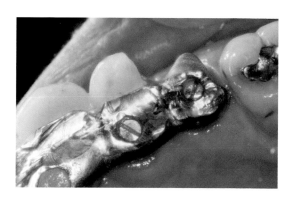

Fig 7-5 A fractured partial prosthesis due to the excessive loading.

85

the generation of excessive stresses in poorly placed prostheses. Partial loss of acrylic or porcelain and fracture of the metal framework is more often than not the result of excessive loading or poor design of the framework. Long cantilevers can lead to both fracture of the prostheses and screw-loosening. As with fracture of any restoration, the cause of the failure must be diagnosed before planning remedial treatment (Fig 7-5).

Loosening or Fracturing of Screws
Overload, poor fit of framework or components and excess or inadequate tightening are all reasons for the loosening or fracturing of screws. Prescribed protocols must be followed to retrieve and replace fractured screws successfully.

Lute Failure in a Cement-Retained Prosthesis
Excessive loading and poor fit of the superstructure are the most common causes for this type of failure. Remedial treatment may include repositioning the superstructure to improve fit. Repeated cement failure may necessitate a remake of the prosthesis.

Fracture or Loss of the Implant
Bone loss may continue to a level at which inherent weaknesses in the implant result in fracture. Excessive loading may result in loss of integration. Further treatment under such circumstances is highly dependent on the particulars of the case. Removal of a fractured implant may be problematical.

Physiological Problems

Physiological problems may include:
- soft-tissue inflammation - peri-implant mucositis and peri-implantitis
- bone loss resulting in implant thread exposure – depending on severity bone loss may necessitate implant replacement
- loss of integration – implant removal and perhaps replacement.

Maintenance

The importance of a carefully planned, fully adhered-to maintenance programme cannot be overemphasised in the long-term management of implant-retained prostheses. In the assessment and treatment-planning of implant cases, it is essential that patients take responsibility for the long-term care of their prostheses. A degree of dexterity will be needed for the patient to clean the prostheses adequately, and this must be carefully assessed

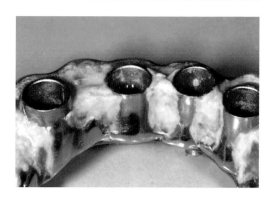

Fig 7-6 The undersurface of a full arch prosthesis showing extensive collection of plaque and calculus.

at the treatment-planning stage. Failure or the inability of patients to maintain and look after their implant-retained prostheses may lead to many varied problems, including failure in clinical service.

It is essential that baseline radiographs are taken at completion of treatment. Most implant systems show a small amount of bone loss in the first year after loading, but should remain stable thereafter. Progressive bone loss may be related to excessive loading. It is therefore recommended that all patients be seen three months after the completion of treatment, when careful clinical examination is indicated. This should include:

- assessment of the prosthesis
- examination of the soft tissues
- radiographic examination to assess bone height.

The Prosthesis

Clinical examination of the prosthesis should - in addition to checking fit, stability, occlusal relationship and patients acceptability - focus on the sufficiency of the patient's oral hygiene. There are numerous aids that can be used to clean around the prosthesis and implant abutments. These range from conventional to electric toothbrushes, floss and super floss and various interdental brushes and related devices. The patient should be encouraged to maintain a high level of oral hygiene around the prosthesis and receive detailed oral hygiene instructions (Fig 7-6).

The Soft Tissues

Evaluations of soft tissues surrounding implant abutments should be both systematic and detailed. Gentle probing should not result in bleeding or exu-

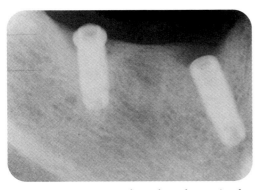

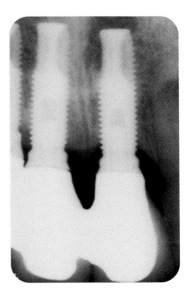

Fig 7-7 (top) Fractured implant due to inadequate number of implants supporting a large prosthesis.

Fig 7-8 (right) A one-year follow-up radiograph showing bone loss to the first thread.

date. A standard periodontal probe may be used to evaluate probing depths. This will depend on the thickness of the original mucosa. Any overgrowth of soft tissue or any loss of attachment that may have occurred will result in increased probing depths. Most inflammatory conditions can be managed by careful attention to oral hygiene, aided and supported by professional advice and assistance. Any deposits that have built up must be removed by the practitioner or by a trained hygienist. There are numerous instruments available on the market to aid removal of any hard deposits around implants. These may be of plastic or carbon-reinforced designs. The use of ultrasonic and metal-tipped scalers is contraindicated.

Long-cone radiographs should be taken:
- at baseline on completion of treatment (Fig 7-7)
- at three months and one year postoperatively (Fig 7-8).

If there is radiographic evidence of bone loss during the first year in clinical service, subsequent radiographs should show very little change. Progressive bone loss is not usually associated with implant-retained prostheses. Any progressive bone loss should be cause for concern and encourage the practitioner to assess the sufficiency of the prostheses.

Soft-tissue inflammation (mucositis) is sometimes seen around poorly maintained and loose prostheses. If the prosthesis is loose it will be necessary to

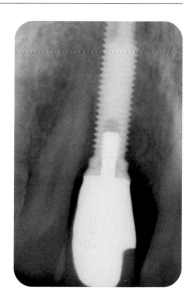

Fig 7-9 A radiograph showing bone loss to the sixth or seventh thread, suggesting excessive loading.

remove it, clean it in an ultrasonic device and securely replace it in the mouth. Soft-tissue proliferation may occur around poorly designed and ill-fitting superstructures. If such proliferation does not respond to local oral hygiene measures it may be necessary to excise the unwanted tissue, possibly as part of remedial treatment to replace the superstructure with an appropriately designed, well-fitting prosthesis.

Peri-implantitis – a peri-implant inflammatory condition resulting in progressive bone loss – is a rare occurrence in well executed and maintained cases. Diagnosis of peri-implantitis may be confirmed by means of long-cone radiographs (Fig 7-9).

Bone loss is usually circumferential, resulting in 'gutter bone loss'. The cause of peri-implantitis is not fully understood, but it may be a combination of excess of or inappropriate occlusal forces in the presence of pathogenic bacteria in an unfavourable oral environment.

The management of peri-implantitis involves:
- careful assessment of the occlusion in the intercuspal position and eccentric movements
- examination and cleaning of exposed implant surfaces. If there has been tissue proliferation around the implants, this may need to be removed

- removal, cleaning and servicing of the restorations as may be indicated clinically
- instruction of the patient in effective oral hygiene procedures
- monitoring and further oral hygiene and prostheses maintenance instruction as necessary.

If peri-implantitis persists and progresses despite the above measures, the case should be critically reviewed and, if required, the patient referred for specialist care.

Conclusions

Complications are rare and fall into two main groups — surgical and prosthodontic. The practitioner should be fully aware of any possible complications prior to treatment and inform the patient accordingly. The cause of prosthodontic complications should be carefully assessed, diagnosed and rectified. The maintenance of implant patients should include regular reviews involving radiographic examinations.

Further Reading

Renouard F, Rangert B. Risk Factors in Implant Dentistry – Simplified Clinical Analysis for Predictable Treatment. London: Quintessence Publishing, 1999.

Chapter 8
The Future

Aim

The aim of this chapter is to give a brief overview of anticipated developments in the use of existing implant systems.

Outcome

Having read this chapter, the reader should be aware of the need to keep abreast of developments in implantology.

Introduction

The future of implant dentistry is clearly exciting. With the further development of systems and techniques implantology may be anticipated to have a major impact in most aspects of dentistry. Some key areas are listed below.

Paediatric Dentistry

The role of dental implants in the management of younger patients is limited, given that implants should not normally be placed until the cessation of growth. While implant dentistry, as we know it today, may not be able to add a great deal to paediatric dentistry, aspects of paediatric dentistry can do a great deal to facilitate implant treatments in patients reaching adulthood, for example:
• space maintenance
• the retention of traumatised teeth with poor prognosis through to adulthood (Fig 8-1).

Orthodontics

The link between implant dentistry and orthodontics is two-fold:
• In space creation, the orthodontist must be fully aware of the room required to place an implant.
• Implants may be used by the orthodontist as a form of anchorage in selected, advanced cases (Fig 8-2).

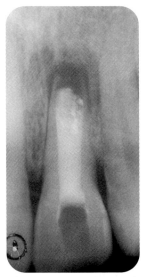 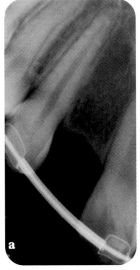 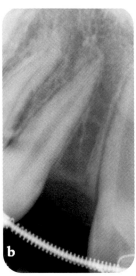

Fig 8-1 A radiograph showing a traumatised tooth filled with calcium hydroxide to maintain alveolar bone.

Fig 8-2 (a) Preoperative and (b) postoperative orthodontic radiographs showing a space created to receive an implant.

Restorative Dentistry

We have considered the value of implants in replacing teeth. The challenge to the profession now is to weigh up the long-term benefits of implants against other forms of prosthodontics and, in particular, saving teeth at all costs.

Periodontics

There is sometimes a tendency to resort to implant dentistry when all else has failed. The question for the future is: Should teeth be removed at an early stage of progressive periodontitis in an endeavour to maintain bone levels, in contrast to years of periodontal treatment that may result in inadequate bone for implant placement? The relationship between susceptibility to periodontal disease and implant failure remains to be resolved (Fig 8-3).

Endodontics

Implants offer a further treatment option to the endodontist in managing teeth of poor prognosis. High levels of success can be achieved with present-day instrumentation and endodontic techniques. Unfortunately, remaining tooth

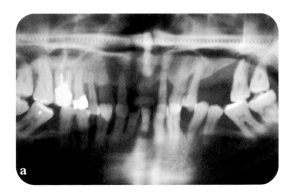

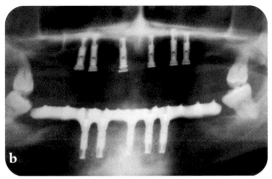

Fig 8-3 (a) A dental panoramic radiograph of a young patient with extensive periodontitis (b) Same patient with lower arch following reconstruction and implants in the upper arch awaiting second-stage treatment.

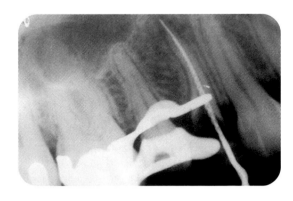

Fig 8-4 Periapical radiograph of a tooth of poor prognosis undergoing root canal therapy.

structures may fail, regardless of endodontic success (Fig 8-4). As with periodontology the question that needs answering in relation to teeth of poor prognosis is when to treat and when to replace with an implant.

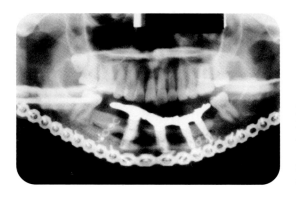

Fig 8-5 A dental panoramic radiograph of a patient with extensive bone grafting and the use of implants following removal of an osteosarcoma of the mandible.

Maxillofacial Surgery and Prosthodontics

The treatment of maxillofacial defects has been transformed by developments in implantology. Applications for implants in this field continue to expand (Fig 8-6).

Education

It is now possible to adopt a team approach to implant dentistry, and dental education should reflect this at all levels, ensuring that all members of the dental team can extend the application of implant dentistry for the benefit of the patients.

Any practitioner wishing to get involved in implant dentistry needs to invest time and effort to acquire the necessary skills and gain a full understanding of the subject area. The level of involvement is up to the individual, but a basic knowledge of implants is vital when discussing treatment options with patients. Practitioners can then either refer the patient for part or all of the treatment. However, many practitioners are comfortable with the restorative aspects of implant treatment and elect to refer patients for surgical phases of treatment only.

Research

Recent developments in implants have included modifications to surfaces to enhance osseointegration. Efforts will continue to make the osseointegration process quicker and even more predictable. Research is ongoing for alternatives to the use of autogenous bone taken from donor sites in the patient. The areas include enhancing bone growth with plasma-rich platelets, the use of bone morphogenic proteins. Further research into ceramic-based implants and implant longevity and cost benefits is set to continue.

Challenges

The limitations of implant dentistry currently include the complexity of the procedures, the large number of components and initial set-up costs. The challenge, therefore, to the manufacturers for the future is to:
• simplify and rationalise the components and their use
• maintain predictable success rates
• reduce start-up costs.

The continued success of implants may challenge many more conventional approaches to dental care, and it is therefore important for the young practitioner, in particular, to be competent and keep up to date in implant dentistry. This book is only an introduction. Further reading has been suggested at the end of selected chapters.

Conclusions

Implants have a role in the various disciplines of dentistry. Education is the key to knowledge and vital to successful treatment. As science leads to further development, continued professional education is essential to maintain a high standard of patient care.

Index

Quintessentials for General Dental Practitioners Series
in 36 volumes

Editor-in-Chief: Professor Nairn H F Wilson

The Quintessentials for General Dental Practitioners Series covers basic principles and key issues in all aspects of modern dental medicine. Each book can be read as a stand-alone volume or in conjunction with other books in the series.

Publication date, approximately

Oral Surgery and Oral Medicine, Editor: John G Meechan

Practical Dental Local Anaesthesia	available
Practical Oral Medicine	available
Practical Conscious Sedation	available
Practical Surgical Dentistry	Autumn 2005

Imaging, Editor: Keith Horner

Interpreting Dental Radiographs	available
Panoramic Radiology	Autumn 2005
Twenty-first Century Dental Imaging	Spring 2006

Periodontology, Editor: Iain L C Chapple

Understanding Periodontal Diseases: Assessment and Diagnostic Procedures in Practice	available
Decision-Making for the Periodontal Team	available
Successful Periodontal Therapy – A Non-Surgical Approach	available
Periodontal Management of Children, Adolescents and Young Adults	available
Periodontal Medicine: A Window on the Body	Autumn 2005

Implantology, Editor: Lloyd J Searson

Implantology in General Dental Practice	available
Managing Orofacial Pain in Practice	Spring 2006

Endodontics, Editor: John M Whitworth

Rational Root Canal Treatment in Practice	available
Managing Endodontic Failure in Practice	available
Managing Dental Trauma in Practice	Autumn 2005
Preventing Pulpal Injury in Practice	Autumn 2005

Prosthodontics, Editor: P Finbarr Allen

Teeth for Life for Older Adults	available
Complete Dentures – from Planning to Problem Solving	available
Removable Partial Dentures	available
Fixed Prosthodontics in Dental Practice	available
Occlusion: A Theoretical and Team Approach	Spring 2006

Operative Dentistry, Editor: Paul A Brunton

Decision-Making in Operative Dentistry	available
Aesthetic Dentistry	available
Indirect Restorations	Spring 2006
Communicating in Dental Practice: Stress Free Dentistry and Improved Patient Care	Spring 2006
Applied Dental Materials in Operative Dentistry	Spring 2006

Paediatric Dentistry/Orthodontics, Editor: Marie Therese Hosey

Child Taming: How to Cope with Children in Dental Practice	available
Paediatric Cariology	available
Treatment Planning for the Developing Dentition	Autumn 2005

General Dentistry and Practice Management, Editor: Raj Rattan

The Business of Dentistry	available
Risk Management	available
Practice Management for the Dental Team	Autumn 2005
Quality Matters: From Clinical Care to Customer Service	Autumn 2005
Dental Practice Design	Spring 2006
IT in Dentistry: A Working Manual	Spring 2006

Quintessence Publishing Co. Ltd., London